Go
Get
Him!

About the Author

Avril Mulcahy is Ireland's no. 1 modern matchmaker. Blending traditional matchmaking with modern-day technology, psychology and business know-how, she has helped hundreds of singles find their perfect match. Avril holds a BComm and MA in Public Relations and is also a licensed neuro-linguistic programming (NLP) coach.

Avril's boutique matchmaking agency has successfully matched top CEOs, successful entrepreneurs, farmers, nurses, teachers and lawyers with like-minded partners. Known for her tough love approach, she also has lots of patience, an eye for chemistry and a passion for fun. As a trusted dating coach, her goal is clear – to get people dating. She uses her NLP skills to help singles break the routines, bad habits and attitudes that are holding them back from a dating life that their married friends would be jealous of!

Her matchmaking career began almost 10 years ago when she began organising singles events in Ireland and Australia. She came to national media attention when she launched her own dating experiment, 40 Dates in 40 Days, with an accompanying blog detailing her journey through the Irish dating scene.

Avril frequently contributes to media discussions about love, sex, dating and relationships and has appeared on RTÉ's *The Saturday Night Show*, RTÉ's *Today*, ITV's *This Morning* and TV3's *Ireland AM*, as well as contributing numerous articles on the same subjects to print media, including *The Irish Independent*.

Go
Get
Him!

**Everything you need to know
to create the love you want**

Avril Mulcahy

GILL & MACMILLAN

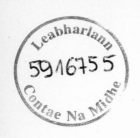

Gill & Macmillan
Hume Avenue, Park West, Dublin 12
www.gillmacmillanbooks.ie

© Avril Mulcahy 2014

978 07171 6524 7

Edited by Kristin Jensen
Design and typesetting by Fidelma Slattery

Printed and bound by CPI Group (UK) Ltd, Croydon, CR0 4YY

This book is typeset in Bembo 11pt on 13.

The paper used in this book comes from the wood pulp of managed
forests. For every tree felled, at least one tree is planted, thereby renewing
natural resources.

A CIP catalogue record for this book is available from the British Library.

5 4 3 2 1

Dedicated to all my fellow goddesses in the world:
from even a little spark may burst a flame.

Contents

Get Ready

Get Set

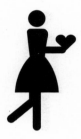

Go!

Acknowledgements

Thank you, thank you, thank you to everyone who helped me make this book possible. The road wasn't always easy, but thank you for helping me find my way, making me buckets of tea, feeding me, listening to me bang on about flames, moths, dickheads and sexual goddesses and giving me the encouragement and sometimes the kick up the arse that I needed to stop faffing and start writing.

Thank you so much to Gill & Macmillan, especially to Deirdre Nolan and Kristin Jensen for working with me directly, understanding my chaotic writing style, stitching it all together and making it all happen. Thank you, ladies. Words cannot express how grateful I am. Just thank you.

Deirdre Rennison Kunz, thank you for putting the final touches on the book. Teresa Daly, from one PR girl to another, you are one of a kind! Thanks for giving me such a great platform so as many people as possible can hear about *Go Get Him!*. Actually, thank you to the entire Gill & Macmillan team and to the designer, Fidelma Slattery. You have provided me with fantastic support that just keeps on giving.

Thanks to all my clients and single friends. Thank you for being so honest, for sharing your dating woes with me and for taking action towards a better dating life. This book is the result of the many conversations, coaching sessions and testimonials I've had with you.

A huge thank you must go to all my family and friends, of course, who make me the kind of person I am today. As Marilyn Monroe said, 'I'm selfish, impatient and a little insecure. I make mistakes, I am out of control and at times hard to handle. But if you can't handle me at my worst, then you sure as hell don't deserve me at my best.' Thank you for being there for me through thick and thin. Thanks to my parents for bringing me into this world, keeping the wolf from the door, educating me and supporting my chosen path even though it didn't fit the norm. Thanks to my brother Jack for being the best brother to me. I'm blessed to have you in my life. Thanks to all my aunties who over the years taught me to be mindful and measured with a bucketful of madness thrown in. Deirdre Lacey, thank you for your fantastic help with just about everything and for being there through it all. You, Miss Dee, are a lady, a legend and a dear friend. And to Elaine Walsh, one of my dating mentors and an all-round goddess, you have taught me valuable life lessons.

Thank you to the Irish Institute of NLP for changing the way I think about life and giving me the foundation to create my own destiny. To the media, thank you for always giving me an opportunity for my voice to be heard, especially to *RSVP* magazine for taking the risk and publishing my monthly column, 'Love Buzz'.

A special thank you to the following friends for all the love, support and great times: Jennifer Muldowney, Margaret Folan, Frank Towey, Sharon D, Arlene McMahon, Rosana Vidal, Tara Miller, Astrid Lawton, Ruth McCormick, Emily Cox, Joey Middleton, Roisin Haughey, Masters of PR Course Director John Gallagher, Catherine Lennon, Grainne Byrne, Pat Flood, Anita Crosse, Paul Hughes, Anthony Kelly, Marianne Doyle, Ian Gamble, Kritika Ashok, Shruthi Chindalur, JP O'Sullivan, Aimee Milne, Lorraine Clifford, Brent Pope, Liz Merriman and all the many men I've dated. I will never forget what you have done for me over the years.

May your lives be filled with health, joy, love and happiness!

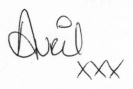

XXX

The Relationship = Happiness Myth

We've all had to face the dreaded question: 'Why are you single?'

You know the awkward silence that follows, where you try to defend your single status without looking like a desperado. You know the kind of crap you get from married women, who within two minutes of meeting you will declare, 'I have a man – do you?' Or perhaps you've judged someone else. Maybe you've thought, 'Well, there must be something wrong with her if she's still single.'

Does this all ring a bell?

A lot of people don't know what to do with you as a single because you don't fit in with what society says you should be. People have this idea from the media or romantic films that if you're in a relationship, you must be happy. In our culture and society, relationships and marriage are associated with success.

I am here to tell you that the equation **1 Male + 1 Female = Happiness** is complete and utter bullshit. A relationship will not make you happy or complete you. Nobody else can make you happy – only you can.

Forget about what society says. Society says a lot of things, but it doesn't always get it right. Society will always have a new notion on how you should live your life. There will always be a new fad on how to be happy.

The goal of this book isn't to be in a relationship by the time you've finished reading it – I would be lying to you if I promised you that. As a professional matchmaker, I have numerous clients coming to me who expect me to work wonders for them. Some women seem to think that I can make a man for them or order him from a catalogue and deliver him to their door. Plenty of women come to me and say they want to find a husband in three months. I would love to be able to do this for my clients, and if I could, I'd already be a millionaire and would be lying on a beach in the Caribbean right now. But life doesn't work like that, and relationships and love definitely don't work like that either. I can't make someone want to be in a relationship with you. I can't make someone want to commit to you. I can't make someone love you.

The goal of this book is to give you the best possible chance to get out there and increase your opportunities to meet great men who you could *potentially* have a healthy relationship with, or a casual fling, or whatever you choose. The book centres around building you into a high-value woman so that your true goddess can shine. Once you figure this out, you will make better choices and you won't put up with the shite that's out there. When you love, nourish and support yourself, then what I *can* promise you is that you will be happy all by yourself. And you know what? That happy person is so attractive to men.

Your *Go Get Him* road map

The book is separated into three sections: 'Get Ready', 'Get Set', 'Go!'.

1. Get ready

'Get Ready' will help you fall in love again with your dating life and your vision of a relationship. Take time to appreciate the brilliance, beauty and magnificence of you, and with my help, decide to make it even better. Never forget that you are one of a kind and great things will happen to you when you take a full hold of your life. I will show you the importance of silencing your own single woman victim mentality and other destructive dating patterns that can steal your joy, harm your dating growth and block you from opportunities to meet great men. Sure, some women have met the man of their dreams with little effort – and some women have also won the lotto. It's time to stop leaving things to chance.

2. Get set

'Get Set' gives you a plan of action to live a better dating life. There are things in your dating life that are no longer working for you, and you know it in your heart. Become more daring and try things that you have never tried before. In this section, I will ask you to challenge yourself and I will show you how to meet more men.

3. Go!

With a firm foundation now in place, the 'Go' section will show you how to get in touch with your inner goddess and put the finishing touches to your dating life so that you can really get out there – wiser, sexier and with a new spring in your step.

Opportunities to meet (OTM)

The dating market is really just like any other market. You're shopping for a great mate. You decide your route to market to advertise your best qualities. It requires an investment of time and cash, but the payoff – love, maybe even a long-term commitment – is priceless. But you need to stop waiting for Prince Charming to come knocking on your door. Many women say they don't want to be alone, but they rarely want to put in the effort it takes to simply find men to date. If you want change, then do something to create change.

The OTM strategy breaks dating down into one simple task: create opportunities to meet men. The OTM strategy gets your networks working for you and shows you how to manoeuvre through them. Keep the OTM strategy firmly at the forefront of your mind as you read this book. You have opportunities all around you right now, and with the right attitude you'll suddenly be surrounded by prospective date possibilities!

40 dates in 40 days

How do I know so much about OTMs? Why am I so convinced that there are so many possibilities out there? Because I did it, and I did it all in 40 days.

As a research project, I set myself a challenge to find a date for every day of Lent. I got dates from online agencies, from singles events, from other matchmakers and from friends. My own mammy even set me up on a date. Did I get a relationship out of the experience? No, but that wasn't the point. In fact, the experiment wasn't even conducive to a relationship, as I knew I had a date with another man the next day. The 40 dates in 40 days project was an intensified version of the OTM strategy. So now, whenever anyone tells me there are no men left, I can simply say that there are, and I got 40 of them in a row.

The law of attraction is a load of rubbish

When I was younger my mother always said to me, 'What's meant for you won't pass you.' I even put that quote on my Bebo page and I was known to say it aloud to anyone in my vicinity for years. I also used to be a fan of *The Secret* – believe it, think it, focus on it. I'm a big believer in positive thinking, but I was thinking, focusing and believing to the point of combustion and nothing was happening for me.

The law of attraction – that you can get positive results simply by thinking about them – is a load of rubbish. You have to be positive, but one of the vital ingredients missing in the law of attraction is the word *action*. Attraction is **attr + ACTION**, and *The Secret* forgot to mention the action part.

One of my clients had read numerous versions of *The Secret* and had a library full of books about attraction. She came to me to seek out my advice as yet another problem-solving game-changer. I suggested that she'd been spending too much time reading books and believing that she could manipulate the universe into motion while sitting on her couch engaged in rigorous attraction thought. She actually admitted as much but had kept doing the same thing – thinking really hard, doing nothing and yet somehow still hoping to find a partner – because it was within her comfort zone. I immediately got down to work drawing up some action points to get her up off her couch and out dating. You won't get anything in life unless you work in an actionable, goal-oriented, committed and accountable way, and that goes for your dating life too.

Dating starts at the end of your comfort zone

Clients often tell me, 'I feel stuck in my dating life and I don't know how to fix it.' Do you feel the same way? You have come to the right place, as this is something I work on when I coach clients.

During the coaching session, we often realise that something has got to change. Your dating life has become stagnant, there are inner frustrations or you are on autopilot in your dealings with men.

So many people date 'comfortably', waiting to meet the same type that just isn't working for them or who doesn't excite them or make them feel loved, sexy, secure, attractive or connected. We often choose to stay within a zone that is familiar to us, one where we know what to expect. Yes, I did say *choose* to stay, because you do have a choice here. To put it another way, what are you saying NO to by choosing to stay inside your comfort zone?

Many of my clients are afraid of dealing with the unknown. Not knowing what to expect is something most of us have to face at some stage in our dating lives. I had one client a while back who said she could never go online. When I asked her why not, she said, 'There are loads of people I don't know on it.' I simply said, 'That's exactly the point!'

When my clients are dealing with unfamiliarity in their dating life and are about to embark on their dating plan, I encourage them to break it down it into small, manageable chunks and make one simple change every day for the first few weeks. If you make one small change every day, in 30 days you will have made 30 changes – that's got to make a difference. For example, on day one you write your online profile, on day two you choose your pictures (this may require more time if you don't already have them), on day three you sign up to an online dating site and on day five you send your first online message. Imagine what could happen if you kept this momentum up. If you keep doing one simple thing to improve your dating life for three months, that's nearly 100 changes to your current dating life. Little by little, you will become more knowledgeable about your new dating world. Each day you will step a little closer to a more fulfilled dating life. Each day you will learn a little more about yourself and become stronger, sexier and more confident in yourself.

Clients who commit to my plan of doing one thing for their dating life every day tell me how their confidence grows, their fear diminishes and how excited they are by the progress they're making. Where once they felt overwhelmed by their dating life or challenged by their prospects or their destructive dating patterns, they now start to see how small, consistent steps taken on a regular basis build a steady momentum and they will start meeting men for sure. When I do the three-month follow-up call, the clients who got outside their comfort zone and are really committed to change always tell me how they feel more confident, are meeting more men and are enjoying the process – with or without a relationship.

The first step is to start moving out of your comfort zone and into one that may initially feel scarier, but in reality it's far more exciting. So what are you waiting for?

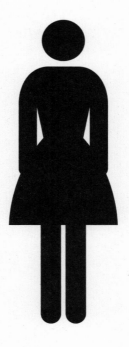

Get Ready

Stop Faffing and Start Doing!

There are lots of indicators that you want to date more. Do any of these apply to you?

- ♥ You feel lonely.
- ♥ You feel isolated.
- ♥ All your friends are married.
- ♥ You feel like your life is missing something or someone.
- ♥ You're sitting in on endless Friday nights on your own.
- ♥ Your cat or dog is becoming your best friend.
- ♥ You've become anti-men and have given in to the single victim mentality.
- ♥ You feel like you're stuck in a dating rut.
- ♥ You haven't had a date in a year.
- ♥ You haven't had sex in over a year.
- ♥ You've had numerous dates but none of them lead anywhere.
- ♥ You don't know what you're looking for.
- ♥ You feel like dating is only for people in their twenties.
- ♥ You're dating someone who you know isn't suitable, but if you break up with him you'll be on your own.
- ♥ You don't know where to start in dating.
- ♥ You don't have enough time to date.
- ♥ You don't meet a lot of men.

Forget about what other people think. Forget about your Auntie Josie giving you the old maid eyes. Forget about your friends gossiping in a small town. Forget about the fact that you might be the last of your friends to get married. You will find someone when it's your time. But the more chances you create for yourself, the more opportunities you have of meeting a like-minded man. I'm going to show you a plan of action to meet more men, but you have to be ready too. All change requires effort, but the more you give, the more your dating life will give back to you.

This book is all about self-awareness, but awareness by itself isn't good enough. Once you become aware of who you are, your dating patterns and your routines, you have to learn how to work with it, and sometimes through it.

The dating wheel

Let's get a quick overview of what point you are at in your dating life. In order to develop good dating habits, you first need to establish where you are now and what isn't working. An assessment of where you are today in your dating life will give you an insight into why you don't have the kind of relationship success you want and it will help you determine what's holding you back. I'm going to throw out a wobbler here – your dating environment might not be the biggest problem. *You* might be the biggest factor in your own dating downfall.

Perfection is not required, and it's not desirable. Start plotting exactly where *you* are now in each of the areas. This will take a few minutes. Ask yourself this question: *Right now, at this very moment, am I waiting or am I creating? Am I taking the positive steps that will give me results in my love life?* If your answer is no, take heart. By reading this book, you are already taking action by trying to make the changes necessary to make progress.

The dating wheel on page 7 will give you a snapshot of your dating life right now. Below is a brief overview of each of the six segments of the wheel. Everyone is different, so make sure your dating wheel is personal to you.

1. Self-esteem

How are you feeling right now? How confident are you about yourself? Perhaps you're struggling to get over a break-up. Perhaps you were brought up in a family who was very critical of you. Perhaps you don't think you're worthy enough to meet a wonderful, relationship-minded man. This section is personal to you.

2. Dating life

Rate yourself on how many dates you have been on in the last 12 months. Give yourself a mark on how happy you are with your dating life.

3. Relationships priority

How much of priority is being in a relationship to you right now? How much time have you put into finding a relationship?

4. Fun and creativity

You might be wondering what fun and creativity have got to do with dating, but research shows that happy people seek out creative tasks, are more likely to be more active, make happiness a priority and seek out the company of other happy people. The best thing about all of this is that the more fun events you go to that incorporate your hobbies and interests, the more chances you are giving yourself to meet someone like you, and boom – the more chances you have of meeting someone.

5. Social

Rate yourself on how happy you are with the social connections in your life. How can you build networks in your work, with your friends and around your hobbies? These connections will all help you in your dating life. We'll talk about this more later on.

6. Packaging

Sorry, ladies, but we live in a visual world and packaging gets a whole segment on the wheel. It's really important that you put down where *you* are now, and not in relation to other people. For example, I'm no Cindy Crawford and I'm never going to be. I'm slim, pale and tall with crazy frizzy hair. I have to work with what I've got. I'd give myself a 6 right now. My hair could with do with colouring, I could stand to lose half a stone so that LBD will get worn at the next wedding and my nails are a bit worse for wear. I try to buy clothes that suit my pear shape, but I'm never going to have Naomi Campbell's skin or Nicole Scherzinger's gleaming silky locks. I'd like to go up to a 7 or 8, as I want to sort out all those points I listed above. But that's personal to me.

EXERCISE:
THE DATING WHEEL

On a scale of 1 to 10, circle where you are in each of the areas. One is the lowest marking and means you are totally dissatisfied with this area. Ten is the highest score and means you are completely happy.

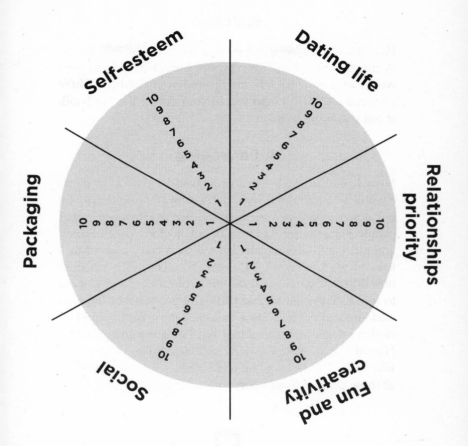

As soon as you finish, plot where you would like to be by the time you finish this book. There's no point plotting where you are now if you aren't going to do anything about it. Remember the reason you bought this book? Your dating life isn't working, so once you know what you need to change, it will set you in motion to make those changes.

EXERCISE: LOOKING TO THE SHORT-TERM FUTURE

Where would you like to be in each of these areas by the time you finish this book?

Self-esteem

How would you like to feel about yourself?

_____

_____

Dating life

What would you like your dating life to look like?

_____

_____

Relationships priority

Would you like to feel more motivation, less motivation or the same amount of motivation towards relationships?

_____

_____

Fun and creativity

What fun and creative activities would you like to have in your life?

_____

_____

Social

What do you want your social life to look like?

....

....

Packaging

How would you like to look?

....

....

Are you a doer or a faffer?

A lot of people come to me and say they are stuck in their dating life. I'm sorry to disappoint you, but you're not stuck – you're what I call faffing. There is no such thing as being stuck. You can be stuck in the mud and you can get stuck in a lift, but you can't get stuck in your mind unless you decide to stay in limbo land. There are always three choices in this world: do it, don't do it, or faff around thinking about doing or not doing it. Are you a doer or a faffer? Let's start doing!

There's an added benefit to taking your dating life into your own hands. When you know that you are doing everything in your power to improve your relationship situation, you can be content even if the results aren't immediate. Simply knowing that you are moving forward in a significant way will make you happier. So let's start moving forward!

First steps

Now that you've finished plotting, you have an overview and some specific targets. You know where you are now and what you can improve to get to where you want to be. So let's make this simple. What are the first steps you can take today – right now – to improve your dating life?

For example, if I felt that my packaging could do with some improvements, I would write down:

1.

Get hair sorted – buy intense conditioner
to control my frizzy mop.

2.

Lose 3lb – don't eat any bread today.

3.

Sort out dress for the races – ring my friend Mags
and ask if I can borrow that hot blue dress
I saw on her last week.

EXERCISE: FIRST STEPS

What can you do today to improve your dating life?

Self-esteem

1. ....

2. ....

3. ....

Dating life

1. ....

2. ....

3. ....

Relationships priority

1. ....

2. ....

3. ....

Fun and creativity

1. ....

2. ....

3. ....

Social

1. ....

2. ....

3. ....

Packaging

1. ....

2. ....

3. ....

Final month

What would you do if you were told that you were being granted one final month to meet a partner, and that after the month was up you would never have the chance again? You would have the same amount of money you've always had, but you would have as much time as you needed – your job would be taken care of and you would have no family ties to worry about. All you would have to do is focus on your dating life.

The aim of the next exercise is to help you focus on your dating life. Using the present tense, write down what you are going to do over the next 30 days to meet your goal of meeting your soul mate.

EXERCISE: FINAL MONTH

What you are going to do over the next 30 days to meet a great man?

....

....

....

....

♥ ♥ ♥

Read what you've written. Is there anything that you could already be doing? Go back to the first steps exercise and begin to take action. Stop faffing and get going!

Future Pacing

I have every kind of person – young, old, overweight, slim, tall, small, you name it – coming to see me. For some, I can see the pain and loneliness on their faces and they are just begging to be helped. Others swan into my office after reading about me in a magazine, looking to meet the matchmaker and thinking there is something glamorous about the whole thing. But I treat everyone the same.

I always start with a client's dating history and ask them to tell me about the last year of their dating life. What I'm really looking for is a number – no excuses, no reasons, no nothing. I just want to know how many dates they've been on in the last 12 months. You can't glamorise a number, it's just a fact. That's why I always dread going to my accountant. I can get carried away thinking I'm blooming amazing when I'm appearing in all the media or I can blame the recession for clients not paying on time, but that's all irrelevant to my accountant, who makes me take a cold, hard look at my income, which is always a rude awakening. It's the same in dating. This number looks you in the face and gets you to take notice. This number is also the result of your patterns and habits, the good and not so good.

Where you are now in your dating life is the result of habits done over and over again. It could be a habit such as overeating, which means you may have put on a bit of weight; drinking too much, which means you keep going home with losers; working so hard that you don't have time to meet someone or you're too stressed out when you do come home from work; or procrastinating to the point where you never actually do anything.

We typically only focus on the short term, the here and now, which doesn't help your future dating life. Having that chocolate bar every night after dinner, getting drunk every weekend and going home with someone who's unsuitable or putting off really getting out there and meeting people might not seem like a big deal right now, but I can tell you that in the future, it will be.

I have clients who are young and carefree who are just starting to focus on their dating life, and then I have clients who have consistently engaged with their dating life in a negative way and are now finding it very difficult as they get older. Let's face it – it can be more difficult to meet someone the older you are. I can help people change any-thing – their style, their habits and even their attitude – but I can't change your age. I can still help people find oppor-tunities, but a lot of people don't realise that if they keep doing the same unhelpful things in the short term, then in the long term they will never reach their goals. It can be a really emotional realisation for some.

A powerful tool in neuro-linguistic programming (NLP) called 'future pacing' can really help you here. I use it with all my clients and I want you to do it now. In the exercise on page 17, I want you to future pace your current dating life, including all your bad habits. Think about what could happen if you were to keep doing your regular bad habits and what impact it could have on your future dating life in one year, five years and 10 years' time.

In the 'Your future dating life' column, I want you to be as negative as possible. I know this is a dreadful exercise, but

I want to show you what will happen if you keep doing what you're doing now. Nobody wants to talk about the negative thing, the little thorn that's prodding you that you've decided to ignore, saying that it's all fine and every-thing will work out in the end. This fantasy is ruining your dating life and not giving you any motivation to change your patterns, to do something about it and get out there. You need to acknowledge that your negative dating pat-terns are having a negative result, not just now, but also in the future. Think about it this way: let's say your bad dating habit is to procrastinate and you decide to stay in and put off dating for yet another Friday night. But if you knew that if you stayed at home you would miss out on meeting a great guy and never have a date again, would you still choose to stay in? Of course not!

But that's the whole point of this exercise. Because we don't often experience a negative effect immediately in the short term, we don't really see the impacts of some of our bad or unproductive habits. But when they are all added together and compounded over time, it can be a totally different story.

So here's something you can do about it. First you need to identify some of your habits that aren't working or serving you and admit that they are in fact bad habits. Here are a few to help you, but think of five of your own and write them down on the next page.

- ♥ I don't make time for dating and tend not to go out much.
- ♥ I don't put effort into what I wear and tend to wear the same thing when I go out.
- ♥ I have weight up at the moment, so I'm waiting until I lose that until I go back out there again.
- ♥ I spend most of my time with my married friends.
- ♥ I drink a lot of alcohol when I'm out and tend to go for dickheads.

- ♥ I don't meet many men on a weekly basis.
- ♥ I don't generally talk to men on a night out.
- ♥ I don't go on dates because I haven't been focusing on my dating life.
- ♥ I'm often stressed in work and I don't have the energy to invest in my dating life.
- ♥ I talk about work a lot when I'm out.

EXERCISE: MY BAD DATING HABITS

1. ....

2. ....

3. ....

4. ....

5. ....

Now write down your age one year, five years and 10 years from now (yes, that time will come!). Think about what could happen if you continue doing these bad habits over a longer period of time. Write down what your dating life will be like if you still have the same dating habits and the same number of dates that you have now. Step into your future self and tell me about that person. Describe how that makes you feel. Are you lonely? Are you happy? Are you frustrated? Are you angry? It may be the way you are feeling right now, but don't ignore these feelings. Don't bury these feelings and tell yourself it's okay. It's not okay, is it? I know this is difficult and that you might not want to go to this place, but I promise this will help you and motivate you to create change.

	Your age	Your future dating life	How does that make you feel?
1 year from now			
5 years from now			
10 years from now			

I'm sure this exercise was an eye-opener for you, and I'm sure it was painful to step into that place. But this pain is an incredible motivation. Your quest to remove this pain or the perception of your future pain can powerfully push you towards action to create change in your life so that your dating life never ends up like the life you've imagined above.

Now every time you are about to do one of your five bad habits, use these negative mental images to stop you in your tracks and help you consciously choose what you want to do instead. So the next time you're thinking of staying in on your own on a Friday night, think of yourself one year from now, five years from now and 10 years from now. Are your actions today helping that person?

It's not all bad, though! You can also apply the future pacing technique in a positive way. Each and every small positive step or action you take will move you forward and help you grow. Even though it may not instantly get you your desired results (remember, I can't promise you a relationship), actually doing it rather than just thinking about it means that all those small things will add up to make a real difference for your future dating life.

If you don't have a plan for how you want your dating life to be and you aren't doing anything about it, you can bet that things won't end up the way you want. Have you been making the most out of dating life? Can you say you've been doing the best that you can to make the most of yourself and the opportunities around you? Because if you can't, it's time to change things and change your habits so that whether or not you are in a relationship, you can look back on your dating life and smile.

The pull spectrum

Let's talk about the pull-based motivation to create change in your dating life. Even though it's helpful, it's not good enough to just establish the pain as a reason to change. You need to take action not just to remove a current pain, but to bring yourself closer to a deeply desired end. With dating, you know that you can't have a blind ambition that you will definitely get married or definitely find someone who meets all your criteria. As you know, there's no such thing as perfection. But you have to wholeheartedly believe that there is a great, desirable man out there who wants you and you must keeping going until you find him. The mere experience of moving along the 'pull spectrum' to a better dating life, regardless of whether or not you actually hit the relationship quest you're working towards, can be immensely rewarding in and of itself. And this is the mindset that I want you to have – one of full engagement, joy and action.

Are You an Eagle or a Chicken?

Anthony de Mello was a mystic Jesuit priest and therapist who wrote many books and led seminars. My own mother still has a tattered, well-read, underlined copy of his most famous book, *Awareness*, on her bedside table. She was always quoting bits from his book depending on my issue in life. The following passage was taken from another book of his, *Song of the Bird*:

> *A man found an eagle's egg and put it in a nest of a barnyard hen. The eaglet hatched with the brood of chicks and grew up with them.*
>
> *All his life the eagle did what the barnyard chicks did, thinking he was a barnyard chicken. He scratched the earth for worms and insects. He clucked and cackled. And he would thrash his wings and fly a few feet into the air.*
>
> *Years passed and the eagle grew very old. One day he saw a magnificent bird above him in the cloudless sky. It glided in graceful majesty among the powerful wind currents, with scarcely a beat of its strong golden wings.*

The old eagle looked up in awe. 'Who's that?' he asked.
'That's the eagle, the king of the birds,' said his neigh-
bour. 'He belongs to the sky. We belong to the earth –
we're chickens.' So the eagle lived and died a chicken, for
that's what he thought he was.

How does this story make you feel? Are you an eagle or a
chicken?

I share this story because each of us is the golden eagle
and each of us deserves a golden relationship. I know that
sounds like fantasyland, but it's true! The biggest obstacle
to achieving success is our own self-limiting beliefs.

For daters, especially those who have been a casualty of
a few dating wars or whose dating experiences are filled
with frustration, disappointment and perhaps failure, you
can see how easy it would be to distort what is true and
possible while creating many self-limiting beliefs.

But you have whinged enough! You have waited long
enough! You have got to get out there and create change in
your dating life. It's better to be an eagle just for one day
than to be a chicken all your life. Say it with me: I am tired
of being lonely. I am tired of being sad. I am tired of having
a poor dating life. I am tired of meeting bad eggs hoping
that something might happen. It's time to change my dating
life, to live my life, my way! To pursue the relationship that
I want! To celebrate me as the confident, sexy, strong, fun,
independent woman that I am! Starting today, I'm going to
date to the fullest!

Breaking free from these negative beliefs is one of the
most important steps in reaching your goals and achieving
success in dating. As you start to surrender your negative
patterns, beliefs and resentments with your dating life, you
begin to understand that you are really quite free now –
free to create your own opportunities.

What's your excuse?

Below are the typical reasons cited by the hundreds of singles I have worked with. Tick the ones that apply to you and add some of your own.

EXERCISE: LIMITING BELIEFS

☐ I have a fear of rejection.

☐ Nobody wants to date a divorcée.

☐ Nobody wants to date a widow.

☐ Nobody wants to date someone over 40.

☐ I'm demotivated.

☐ I'm bad at keeping to a plan.

☐ I keep going for the wrong guys.

☐ Men keep treating me badly.

☐ I can't travel to meet someone.

☐ I'm bad at dating.

☐ I can't flirt.

☐ I'm not a people person.

☐ I have a fear of relationship difficulties.

☐ I have low self-esteem.

☐ I'm not confident.

☐ I don't have time.

Are You an Eagle or a Chicken?

- ☐ I don't know what I want.
- ☐ I feel inadequate.
- ☐ I procrastinate.
- ☐ I have family issues.
- ☐ I have job issues.
- ☐ There are no single men.
- ☐ Nobody wants me.
- ☐ I'm too fat.
- ☐ I'm ugly.
- ☐ Nobody approaches me.
- ☐ I don't have any energy.
- ☐ Men only like a perfect 8 size and supermodels.
- ☐ All men are cheats and liars.
- ☐ I'm not successful enough.
- ☐ All men online are weird.
- ☐ All men who go to a matchmaker are desperate.
- ☐ I don't want to look desperate.
- ☐ All the good men are taken.
- ☐ Nobody will date me because of my age.
- ☐ Nobody will date me because I'm a single mother.
- ☐ I've tried dating before, but it doesn't work for me.
- ☐ ....
- ☐ ....
- ☐ ....

❤ ❤ ❤

Here are the three most common self-defeating thoughts that I've seen when working with clients.

1. There are no single men

Most of the single women I meet have this limiting belief that there are no single men left. They've all packed up and emigrated to Planet Single Men with no return. And what would all the single men be doing on this planet? Playing football together and drinking beer on their own with no sexual excitement whatsoever? Really? Have you seen *Cast Away*? The poor guy nearly went insane.

Others believe that all men are already in relationships. If that was the case, what would be the point in dating sites, social connection sites, matchmakers and singles events? The dating industry is a billion-dollar business fuelled by single people connecting with each other and online dating sites make their money by helping people to find other singles in their area. Single men do exist!

2. There's nowhere to go to meet single men

The thing I get asked most in my business and in the media is, 'Tell me one place where you can meet a man.' I would love to tell you that you can stay in and finish off that tub of ice cream while waiting for Prince Charming to knock on your door, or that there is a weekly gathering of single men every Tuesday night just around the corner from your house. Some women even think the only place to find eligible men is at the pub (we're in Ireland, after all) and they spend nights on end roaming late-night pick-up joints in search of their lifetime partner.

Unfortunately, there isn't one great place where all the single men congregate. But the good news is that they are everywhere. Great men are all around you.

This morning when you stopped at the coffee shop to get a quick cappuccino, there was a man who noticed you but you were in too much of a rush to notice him. Last week there was a great guy who smiled at you on your way into the gym or who was standing behind you in the queue at the bank, but you were too busy clicking on your phone to see him.

Just like great women, handsome, great men are everywhere. The trick is not to limit yourself by trying to find out where these *men* are, but to create a new attitude and an awareness that you are seen and noticed wherever *you* are.

3. I'm bad at dating

Many singles decide that they are bad daters. Many become so frustrated at being blown off again or meeting yet another jerk that they give up indefinitely and often never date again. Let's face it, some guys – not all – can be real dickheads and use and abuse girls, kicking them to the kerb. That's fact. But some women decide to play out their negative self-fulfilling prophecy that they are bad daters by always going for these loser guys because they think they are the only guys who want them. Still other women say, 'I'm bad at dating, so why even try?'

The dating environment is what it is, so unless you win the lotto tomorrow and can do an invite-only party for all the hot single men out there, you have to manoeuvre through it like everyone else. The dating scene can be difficult. You will meet bad boys and undesirables, you will be rejected, it will be time consuming and you may not meet good-quality guys for a while. But this does not mean that you should give in to your limiting beliefs and settle for a dismal dating life.

Even though you can't change the environment, you *can* create change for yourself by changing your experience, the places you go, how you present yourself and your perspective. People meet people every day. Millions of singles are flirting this very second. You have to stop letting your toxic, limiting beliefs keep you from your chance of a relationship. Creating an objective, balanced mindset will not only help you break the limiting belief cycle and get you out there more, but it also creates a better, more positive state of mind that will help you look more attractive.

The following exercise will help you explore a more supportive inner dialogue rather than letting your thoughts hold you back. It will show you that there is a solution to everything. In the table below, write down all your limiting beliefs on the left-hand side and immediately and objectively write down what the solution could be. This exercise pushes you into fixing the useless beliefs to make them into more useful ones. This is a problem-solving exercise. If you're feeling stuck, it's only because you don't have the skills yet – and that's your solution, so write that down.

Many people allow their dating dream to die because of negative conversations, procrastination, lack of preparation and most of all, from doubt and fear. Hold yourself to higher standards and find solutions that will help you overcome any dating challenge.

Here are a few examples to get you started.

Limiting belief | Solution

Limiting belief	Solution
I'm bad at dating.	I'm going to stop going for bad boys and I'm going to slow down the getting-to-know-you process.
There are no single men left.	There are great guys everywhere and I'm going to find them. I'm going to smile at five men in the supermarket today.

Limiting belief	Solution
All single men online are weird.	There is so much choice online, with so much variety. There are weird people everywhere – pubs, festivals, work and online. I will send some messages this week and get to know a few men online and arrange to meet up.

Fly on

If you really want to break free from your limiting beliefs, you must first become aware of the negative thought patterns that are holding you back. But it's even more important to *act*. The eagle had the ability to fly all along but never even tried. Remember, the more you date, the more you will learn to glide through the dating scene, and like an eagle, your skills will become so sharp that you will quickly spot the duds and fly on.

I Am a Ride

I've been on a mission all my life to find out the secret of attraction. I have worked in the dating industry for the past 10 years, gone to numerous dating seminars and asked match-makers and dating coaches, who all had different answers for me. I even travelled to India to talk to different gurus and wise men to help me solve the attraction conundrum.

On one such trip to India, a wise old man who knew that I was looking for answers recommended that if I stopped this desperate search, the answer would come to me. He said, 'When all things lay in the midst of silence, then there descended onto you from the mighty gurus will be the word.'

So I decided to book myself onto a 10-day silent med-itation retreat to connect with my silent centre. I hoped that this mighty guru would feel sorry for me and raise his head. Ten long, silent days lay before me, just meditation and quiet. On the evening of the tenth day, I met the guru and we sat cross-legged, eyes closed, under a tree in the evening sun. He was the purest, most noble man I had ever been in the presence of. No words passed between us, but I immediately felt a connection with him. It was then that he opened his eyes, looked up and shouted out the secret mantra of attraction.

I got such a fright as he broke our silence. He got up and started to dance around in a frenzy, shouting the attraction mantra from the Himalayan hilltops. This is what I had been waiting for all my life, and it just burst out of him, like a man possessed. He jumped up and down as his voice got louder and louder. It was contagious. Before long, I found myself up on my feet dancing around too, shouting the mantra. Our voices could be heard all over. I felt alive and energised and I wanted to share my experience with everyone.

Do you want to know what it is? You must remember that this mantra, once used, will instantly transform you. Are you okay with that?

I want you to repeat after me, and every time you repeat it, I want your voice to get louder and louder. I want you to believe it. I want you to imagine getting more energised every time you say it. I want you to imagine the mantra seeping into your skin and filling up your entire body all the way to your toes and your fingertips, energising each part of you until you actually become what you are saying, in the same way as the guru did.

Are you ready? Repeat after me:

I

Repeat it again and say it louder:

I

Repeat it again and shout it!

I

Now say:

AM

Now put both words together and shout it:

I AM

Now say the following, and remember the guru shouting it from the hilltops like a man possessed:

A FECKING RIDE

Now put it all together:

I AM
A FECKING
RIDE!

Say it again and again:

I AM A FECKING RIDE! I AM A FECKING RIDE! I AM A FECKING RIDE!

And again, until you truly believe it.

I want you to look in the mirror. I want you to look your reflection in the eyes and tell yourself:

I AM A FECKING RIDE!

The next time you're getting ready for a night out and you're all done up and looking fabulous, look at the mirror and tell the person looking back at you that they are a fecking ride. I want you to shout it, believe it, feel it and know it until you are smiling brightly and ready for your date.

Be a coach, not a critic

Okay, okay, I know that story is pretty far-fetched. But I really did do the 10-day silent camp and I really have spoken to top international dating coaches and read hundreds of books and worked with hundreds of clients at this stage. And throughout my years in the dating game, I have seen one common habit that is detrimental to dating success: so many singles spend too much time criticising themselves, moaning to themselves, complaining to themselves and being nasty to themselves. Then they ask me why men aren't attracted to them. You are telling yourself the most horrid things in the world and you are expecting a man to be attracted to that?

Are you aware of your inner dialogue? Do you often hear a harsh voice in your head telling you not to try to get out there, that nobody wants you? Do you strive to be perfect and won't do anything before you are? If you hold back because you think you're not perfect yet, just think of all the opportunities you will miss out on. The people who are successfully dating are not afraid to try, and believe me when I say that they certainly are not perfect.

When I first met **Sandra**, she was feeling unhappy, stuck in a rut and unable to love herself. During one of our sessions she told me she felt 'fat, ugly and unlovable'. We did a little exercise where I stood Sandra in front of a mirror and asked her what she saw. Her answer was short and definitely sharp: 'A fat, ugly cow that no one would want.' Sandra would literally tell herself this every time she looked in the mirror, so it's not surprising that her self-esteem was at an all-time low.

I asked Sandra to imagine a complete stranger calling her a fat, ugly cow and asked her to respond accordingly. She did so in colourful and inventive language! I then asked Sandra why she was letting her own critic get away with it. The final step for Sandra was to try to picture herself the way those who really loved her did. Did they think she was fat, ugly or worthless? Of course not!

To switch direction, I then asked Sandra to tell me about a time when she felt really good about herself. She told me about being at a wedding five years ago where everyone complimented her about how beautiful and fabulous she looked. She continued to tell me that she felt really sexy that day and could feel men checking her out. Her body language changed towards me and she started to smile as she relived how she felt that day, but for some reason she hadn't thought of it in a long time.

I asked her how she felt now, after reliving that memory. 'Well, I know that I'm fabulous and fun and to be honest I'm a really good friend, but I just need to tell myself that more often.' Amen!

You can change that voice in your head from a critic to a coach. After all, it's your mind and you're the one who's in charge in there. Research has repeatedly shown the power of positive self-talk, which is what most of us call affirmations. Positive affirmations have been used to change behaviour in under-achieving students, heighten athletic performance and have even helped cure diseases. When it comes to social interaction, participants in one study who said self-affirmations before a new social encounter reduced their thoughts about being rejected compared to another group that focused on the party and who would be there.

When you make self-affirmations, you build on positive experiences from the past, and even more importantly, you are programming yourself for new fulfilment in the future. You can be the prime and sole architect of a more sexy and feminine self.

Nicola, 45, came to me because she hadn't been on a date in 12 years. Nicola married her best friend when she was 27 but they separated when she was 33. She had got into a rut of telling herself that nobody wanted her. Even though she was a successful solicitor and had the money to dress well, she had left herself go a little and dressed in drab clothing. She spent every weekend cooped up with her cat watching TV because she felt like a 'washed-up old spinster'.

I asked Nicola to tell me about a time when she had felt like a sexy, feminine, confident woman. She cried, as she could not remember such a moment. She had spent the last 12 years putting herself down and being cruel to herself. Eventually she was able to tell me about a time when she was 19 and full of the joys of life and went to the city for a night out. She wore a black dress, had her hair curled and put on red lipstick. She recalled how all the boys were talking to her and she truly felt like a million dollars. She laughed all night and felt happy and energetic. Nicola smiled as she rediscovered her own beauty and started to step into that 19-year-old self again, something that she hadn't done in a long time.

I asked her to relive that moment in real life and share her experience with me. I got this text from her: 'Hi Avril, I just had to tell you that I'm all dolled up and about to head to that black tie ball and I feel stunning. My sister and I went shopping last week and I bought a sexy black number. Can you believe it?! I will send you a picture. I can't wait for the ball. Should be fun.'

Over the years, Nicola had inadvertently nurtured her inner critic. She allowed that voice to go unchecked, trapping her into living a safe, boring and predictable life that she hated.

Does this sound familiar? By listening to that inner critic, you are robbing yourself of the chance to discover so many things about yourself and what you might enjoy. Sure, you might make an eejit of yourself and you might make mistakes, but isn't that better than sitting in every night with your cat?

Remind yourself that the critic doesn't always tell the truth. You may have things you need to work on – we all do. Acknowledge that you are not perfect – nobody is. If you can change something, like becoming more chatty to the opposite sex, then do it. If you have half a stone to lose, lose it. Don't allow the inner critic to exaggerate your weaknesses enough to stop you in your tracks. We are always moving forward, always evolving and always growing.

Change how you think to change how you feel

Here are a few positive statements to help you in the field of dating:

- ♥ I am confident.
- ♥ I am attractive.
- ♥ I am great fun.
- ♥ I am friendly.
- ♥ Men love me.
- ♥ Men desire me.
- ♥ I am approachable.
- ♥ I love my body, mind and soul.

♥ I am interested in other people.
♥ I am a sexy woman.
♥ I am strong.

If you haven't been feeling any of these statements for a while, think back to times when you did feel confident, approachable, sexy and supported. Recall these events and times in as much detail as possible. What did you see, hear and feel? The fastest way to change how you feel is to change how you think.

You are in charge in your own head. Stop giving yourself such a hard time. Get out of your own way and be good to yourself. After all, you want your date to feel comfortable and good about himself, so why not do it for yourself too? When you are more loving and positive with yourself, you will find that you are more relaxed, more self-confident and more at ease while dating. You will tend to meet more loving guys on the dating scene and will be ready to create a truly fulfilling relationship.

So yeah, the guru story is a bit over the top, but if I sense there's a negative or fearful attitude at the beginning of one my singles event, I usually start with that story and before long the entire group is up on their feet shouting **I AM A FECKING RIDE!** I can guarantee that if you use this, you will feel 100% better about yourself – more sexy, more confident and more fun, which in turn more men will be attracted to.

EXERCISE:
YOUR POSITIVE MANTRA

Using the present tense, write down a positive mantra. Get the engine going until you feel freer and freer to write down whatever comes to mind. Now repeat it every day for the next three months. Feel free to use the examples above.

_____

_____

_____

_____

_____

_____

❤❤❤

Your words create your world, so affirm yourself daily. Monitor your thoughts. What you think about, you bring about, so stay focused on your dating goal. A great guy is right around the corner, so keep moving forward.

♥
Know Your Needs

Abraham Maslow was a renowned psychologist who published a paper back in 1943 that said that in order for a person to survive and thrive, they need to go through a series of stages, or a 'hierarchy of needs'. These needs were placed in a pyramid format, shown on the next page. His theory was that a person has to meet the needs in each category before moving on to the next stage in order to lead a fulfilled life.

So what does this have to do with dating? Well, for a relationship to work, you not only have to meet the needs in each category, but you also have to make sure your potential partner is meeting the criteria too. Let's look at each level in detail and see how it affects how you present yourself to a potential partner and also how you make choices about a potential partner.

HIERARCHY OF NEEDS

Self-actualisation

Morality, creativity, spontaneity, acceptance, experience, purpose, meaning, inner potential

Self-esteem

Confidence, achievement, respect for others, the need to be a unique individual

Love and belonging

Friendship, family, intimacy, sense of connection

Safety and security

Health, employment, property, family and social stability

Physiological needs

Breathing, food, water, shelter, clothing, sleep

Physiological needs – start with the basics

You

Our basic needs are food, water and sleep. If we're deprived of any of these, we become listless, irritable and eventually ill. Just as you're not supposed to go grocery shopping on an empty stomach, never go out hoping to meet someone if you're exhausted from lack of sleep or if you have been abusing your body with either too much or too little food or drink. You're never going to be in the right frame of mind to meet someone or begin a new relationship. If you have a cold or the flu, if you had a bad day in work or a recent bereavement, cancel the date. I'm all about managing your state, but if you're sick, you're sick.

Him

Equally, never go out with a guy who doesn't have the basics right. I'm not going to go into detail here as it's pure obvious, but you'd be surprised by the amount of people who put up with crap.

Safety and security – be secure in yourself

You

This level refers to well-being, both in terms of your health and safety as well as your finances. It boils down to this: be good to yourself. As a coach, I help many women to build up their self-esteem and self-worth. Low self-worth can lead you to make bad dating decisions and take bad risks. Never think that a guy is your only option and never make a decision because you feel desperate. If your self-esteem is low, take some time out of the dating scene for a while and work on building yourself back up again. If you don't love you, how do you expect anyone else to love you? Take some time to fine tune your intuition, trust your gut more, watch for red flags and steer clear of any guy who seems risky.

Being secure and confident is one of the most attractive things in a woman. A woman who isn't secure in her body will lack self-confidence and will ultimately struggle to engage in flirting or in conversation with men. A woman should also be financially secure herself and not look for a man to save her from her maxed-out credit card. Stop looking for a guy to complete you or save you. If you're looking and feeling good about yourself, both on the outside and inside, then it's going to show, you will make good dating decisions and men will find you more attractive.

Him

Make sure your guy is going to give you safety and security. Does he have a job or is he living with his parents? Does he look after his health? Does he have a drink problem? Is he abusive? Is he divorced? If so, how does he talk about his ex-wife? Why did he (or she) leave? Does he talk about friends and family? Does he seem pushy or talk about sex a lot? Does his online dating profile look fake? I know this all sounds basic, but you need to see how socially stable a guy is before a relationship can take place or even before you decide to meet him, so watch for red flags. And remember, if he looks like a duck, walks like a duck and quacks like a duck, he's probably a duck. Your safety needs to come first.

Love and belonging – everyone needs someone to love and to be loved

You

Being able to mix and make friends of either sex, growing to love them and being loved back is essential in order to grow as a person. The more you connect with people, the more you will learn about yourself, the better you will feel about yourself and the more opportunities you will have to meet someone. Having interests and a fun social life will make you more confident and less needy. Surround yourself with people who are supportive and love you. Stay away from anyone who doesn't invest in you or is negative towards you. The happier you are and the more positively you present yourself, the more attractive you will be to men. Makes sense, yeah?

Make sure you have a connection – intellectually, physically and emotionally. Remember that intimacy and sex are part of our needs. That is why flirting and building sexual tension are so important, both at the beginning and in order to keep a relationship alive.

Him

Your potential partner also has a need to feel loved and connected, so make sure the dates aren't all about you and that his feelings, interests and achievements are taken into account. To truly connect with someone, get past the superficial chat that he can get with anyone at all – get inside his soul and try to really understand him. For example, if your date is telling you about a tough day in the office, rather than just saying, 'Want to have a drink and forget about it?', say something like, 'Aw, poor you. Why don't I get you a drink so you can relax and tell me all about it?' In that simple sentence, you've shown him that you really care and have given him an opportunity to open up. You could also add a playful pat on his arm, which again will induce that chemical connection.

Self-esteem – respect yourself and others

You

I can't stop banging on about self-esteem. It's everything. You can never do enough work on building your self-esteem, as everything flows from it. It's just so important to respect yourself and treat other people the way that you would like to be treated, and this is especially true in dating. By showing that you respect yourself and the people around you, guys will see you as a high-valued woman and a bit of a challenge. When you have great self-esteem you will naturally attract all sorts of people into your life, and in doing so you will add such wonderful things to other people's lives – and specifically to a partner's.

Him

Is he showing you respect? Do you have to wait for ages to get a text reply back? Or does he just text you late on a

Sunday night with the message 'I'm bored, how's you?' Is he asking you out or are you constantly chasing him? Does he compliment you or put you down? In short, does he add to your self-esteem or make you feel bad?

He might look like Brad Pitt, but do you want the same things in life? You can play around with this when you're in your twenties, but if you're looking for a relationship and he isn't investing in you and showing you love, then don't look twice at him, no matter how physically irresistible he might seem. In order to get your needs met, stop going for the guys who are all looks but who detract from your self-esteem or make you feel insecure. Lose the risky, heart-racing affairs or the big spenders who will just treat you like a possession for the man who invests in you, makes you feel good and who has the same mindset as you in terms of what you want from life.

If you've ever been stood up or someone promised to call you and didn't, then you'll understand where I'm coming from. This is just basic respect, and not getting it goes against the needs of a high-valued woman – which you are.

Self-actualisation – reaching your full potential

You

Nobody's perfect. Maslow put this stage in last so that once you have fulfilled all of the other stages, you can be open to the world around you and on a continuous path of personal development and learning. Keep referring to your dating wheel and know that you are always evolving. Openness to learning is one of the most attractive traits in someone.

Him

You're interested in ballet and he's into football. So what? Don't rule someone out just because you don't have the same interests. Are you open to learning about each other's hobbies? Can you learn about each other's strengths and weaknesses so that you can both enjoy them and complement them? Relationships are difficult, so there will always be times when you need to check in with yourself to see if you can handle something better. Every couple needs the courage to grow.

Get the basics right

In essence, if we look at what Maslow says in terms of dating, you have to get the basics right in yourself and in a potential partner before a relationship can take place. So decide now to rule out bad boys with addiction, money or abusive issues and anyone who shows any signs of red flags.

But even more importantly, you can't have a healthy relationship with others unless you have a healthy relationship with yourself. It could be said that someone who is happy with their life and who is meeting their own basic human needs might subconsciously give off the right vibes, and a potential partner who is also happy and in the right mindset might pick up on those vibes and there's a spark.

Getting Back to Business: SWOT Yourself

Let's get back to business – literally. In the corporate world, businesses spend thousands of euros to go off on fancy retreats and bring in top coaches and performance experts to determine what the firm's strengths, weaknesses, opportunities and threats are – **SWOT**. This analysis allows a business to think through their situation and make good decisions for their future. It's an incredibly useful technique that helps companies figure out their competitive advantage, exploit the opportunities and diminish any threats before they happen.

I've been doing a **SWOT** analysis on myself for years to give me clarity. It quickly gets me motivated to move forward and it allows me to check in with myself to see what else I can learn and where I can grow. The best thing about **SWOT** is that it's balanced. It's a quick-fire reality check of the good, the bad, the fantasy and the potential threats.

Now imagine if we applied this same concept to dating.

Imagine if we looked at our dating lives and ourselves with an equal balance of reflection and critical awareness. Doing a **SWOT** analysis of your dating life can give you a clear picture of who you are. It also helps you figure out what partner might best suit you, what dating opportunities are around you and even the changes you need to make to avoid any future threats.

One of the reasons that businesses hire outside consultants is because they don't have an emotional connection to the decision-making process. People within the business are emotionally connected and therefore find it harder to see all of their weaknesses and spot the threats. They might also miss obvious strengths because they think they're unexceptional or normal or they miss potential opportunities that are as clear as day to outsiders. The same is true for you as an individual, especially when it comes to your dating life. Many of your strengths are probably things that you think come naturally to everyone. For example, maybe you're a very positive influence on others. You may not realise that your positivity is exceptional and that it's actually a significant strength. In order for **SWOT** to do its job, you need to take your emotions out of the equation and become an outside observer of your dating life.

The benefits of constructive feedback

This is a good time to ask your friends, family and co-workers to share their perspectives on you and to give you feedback on things like your interpersonal skills, your dating patterns (what type of guys you keep going for) and your visual packaging – a scary thought for some. A lot of people hate feedback, but I have to say I love it. Some of my best friends are the people who are willing to tell it to me straight and tell me ways I could do things better. Sometimes your friends don't want to hurt your feelings, so they say nothing. But isn't it better to know that those cropped leggings make your arse look fat rather than being told that you look great in anything?

Ask your supportive group of friends, family and co-workers for feedback on you. Words associated with getting constructive feedback are *helpful*, *productive*, *valuable*, *practical* and my personal favourite, *useful*.

So let's start to **SWOT** your dating life! There is no right or wrong answer here, but you need to be as honest as possible. Once you get all of this down on paper, you'll be able to see your dating life more clearly and it will get you motivated to make changes.

1. Define your goals

Before you start your **SWOT** analysis, you need to know what your goals are. Do you want to find a boyfriend? Date a ton of men? Just have sex? Only you know what kind of a relationship you want. Write it down here.

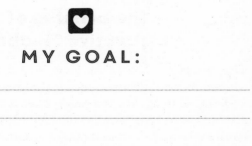

2. Look at your dating strengths

What do you have going for you? What attributes do you have that will help you meet men? What are your strong points in approaching men, dating and relationships? What resources and assets do you have at your disposal? What are you good at when it comes to dating? What have you mastered?

Take note of the things you're good at and your strong points. It's important to identify these and use them to your advantage. Are you good at visually presenting yourself? Are you a good flirt? Are you chatty? Do you meet a lot of men? Do you have great networks? Do you have enough money to invest in dating at the moment? Is age on your side? What do people usually say about your looks? What's your best asset – your eyes, your hair, your smile, your curves? Ask your friends to list your qualities and be kind to yourself.

3. Look at your dating weaknesses and areas that you need to improve

This could be a lack of motivation or something that is holding you back from reaching your full potential. Do you find male company difficult? Do you have limited networks? Have you let your style get outdated or is your hair looking a bit worse for wear at the moment? Again, ask your supportive friends and family for critical and constructive feedback.

You need to be honest here. If you think you've put on a few pounds in the last few years, admit it and write it down. If you feel that you go in for one-night stands too much, own up to it. Start to become aware of your negative patterns. Do you have a weakness for a particular type of guy who usually ends up dumping you? Do you continuously chase men and bombard them with texts and messages? Do you think that you have lots of male friends but no romantic relationships? Is confidence an issue? Do you have issues around commitment? Does your social circle keep you from meeting men?

Write down as much as you can here. Once it gets written down, it will get you motivated to change it. Remember, you're only looking at your dating life here. If career or family stuff comes up, refocus back to your dating life only right now.

4. Look at your dating opportunities

Now use your strengths and weaknesses to consider opportunities and threats. Remember that strengths tend to lead to opportunities and weaknesses tend to lead to threats.

For example, if one of your strengths is that you're a really good friend and are good at one-to-one conversation, an opportunity might be spending more time online, as you get to know men more on a one-to-one basis there. Likewise, if a weakness is that you have put on a few pounds over the last few years, then a threat could be that men will go for slimmer girls.

Once you identify your weaknesses and threats, find out ways to make some needed improvements. Then find ways to focus more on your strengths than your weaknesses. For example, where is opportunity presenting itself? Is there a local club or group you can join? What places have you not been going to to meet new men? Is there already a man in your life who you have a bit of a thing for?

Recognise men and places that you haven't been capitalising on and give it a shot. Did an old fling show up in your life again? Did a new man move into the apartment down the hall?

Is there a new volunteer group or sports club you could join to meet new people? Are there any opportunities arising out of your weaknesses? For example, could you even join a class to help you with one of your weaknesses?

5. Look at your dating threats

What is a potential threat in your dating life? What external roadblocks are stopping you from achieving your goals? For example, do you foresee meeting fewer men at work soon, maybe because you're starting a big project that will take up a lot of your time? Could your habit of comfort eating threaten your visuals? Could being alone for so long mean you're getting more set in your ways? Do you have friends who hold you back? Write it all down in the table on pages 52–53.

Here's an example to help you get started.

Goal:

I want a relationship with a great man who is interested in sports, lives within a two-hour drive, is 30 to 40 years old and has a stable job.

Strengths

- Friends say my smile is my best asset.
- I'm a good listener and I like to ask people questions.
- My friends say that I'm very loyal.
- I like to try new things.
- I'm thoughtful.
- I'm persistent – if I get a goal into my head, I will keep going until I've given it my all.

Weaknesses

- Sometimes I don't know what to say to men.
- I've been spending a lot of time at work recently.
- I need to lose a stone.
- My highlights are growing out.
- My last three boyfriends haven't lasted longer than two months.
- I've only gone on two dates in the last six months.

Strengths

- I'm quite feminine and I like to look after my appearance.
- I like to make people at ease.
- I'm confident when you get to know me and with my friends. My friend Sarah said that I'm always the one with the best story and I'm the most fun to be around.

Opportunities

- When I lose the weight, I can fit into my sexy black dress again and wear it out. I always get loads of attention when I wear it.
- My friend Sarah is an accountant and has said she will invite me out with her next Friday.
- A lot of people seem to be using the online agencies these days. I'm going to sign up and give it a whirl.
- My positive attitude is addictive and people will want to talk to me.
- The next time I'm out, I'm going to start chatting to men rather than just the girls.
- If I like a guy I meet, I'm going to ask for his business card or offer mine.
- I've been told that lots of men go to the local races.

Weaknesses

- I don't have the money to invest in matchmaking at the moment.
- When I'm out, I usually just catch up with the gossip with the girls.
- I can be a little shy at first.
- I sometimes put others' needs first.
- I find it difficult to be tactile with men.
- Men don't approach me.
- I have a tendency to be clingy.
- I meet men but I never swap numbers with them.
- I hate first dates – I get so nervous.

Threats

- My biological clock is ticking. Some men want girls in their twenties.
- My work will get busier, so I'll have less time to invest in dating.
- If my workload increases, I might eat more ready-made meals and hence put on some weight.
- A lot of my friends are getting married this year, so a lot of my time will be taken up going to their hen parties (too many women, not enough men!).
- My friends are all settling down, so I have fewer women to go out with.
- I'm afraid I'll look desperate the older I get.

In short, by giving yourself a **SWOT** analysis, you will be able to:

1.
Identify and utilise your dating strengths

2.
Notice and improve on your dating weaknesses

3.
Recognise and explore some potential dating opportunities

4.
See what threats are standing in your way and holding you back from achieving dating success

EXERCISE: MY SWOT ANALYSIS

My goal:

....

....

....

....

....

Strengths

Weaknesses

Opportunities

Threats

6. Apply the findings

After you have developed a thorough list and filled in your grid, you need to look for ways to apply your findings. You can start by asking questions about each section. For example, how can you use your strengths to make sure you get the most out of each date? In the example above, I'm surprised that so many people who are usually so confident in work or in social scenarios with their friends clam up on dates.

Ask yourself how you can work on your weak areas. How can you exploit each opportunity by using your strengths and make them action points? How can you protect yourself from threats? For example, if you see younger ladies who appear to be more attractive and con-fident than you as a threat because they're snatching up all the good guys, then you need to consider how you can protect yourself from that possibility. Perhaps you need to get a new younger-looking haircut or maybe you need to think about dating guys who are a few years older than you.

The answers to these questions will help you set new goals and new strategies for achieving them. So get to work!

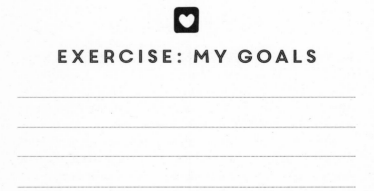

EXERCISE: MY GOALS

MY STRATEGIES FOR ACHIEVING THOSE GOALS:

_____

_____

_____

_____

_____

_____

♥♥♥

At the end of this process, you should have a much clearer idea about who you are, what opportunities you need to pursue and what growth lies ahead. Use this to set goals for the future, clarify your existing goals and get you off your ass to increase your skills and improve your presentation.

SWOT your date

We learned how to **SWOT** your own dating life to get you to take a look at yourself and your dating environment. Now it's time to flip it around – if you've had three or four dates with a guy and it has some potential, then you might want to do a **SWOT** analysis on your date.

In the beginning, we have a tendency to only see a guy's strengths and forget his weaknesses. I'm here to tell you that dating – and life – are not like that. No man is perfect and no man deserves that godlike status. I see so many women putting all their eggs in one basket and booking a one-way ticket to fantasyland after just one date. On the other hand, you can miss some great guys because you weren't open to their strengths.

This exercise will get you to take an objective view of whether or not this guy is actually into you. Is he just throwing you crumbs or is he genuinely looking for the same thing as you?

Apply the same evaluation method of strengths, weaknesses, opportunities and threats. The following questions can help you do that.

Here's an example to show you what I mean by **SWOTting** your date.

Strengths

- ♥ Confident
- ♥ Tall, dark and handsome
- ♥ Very successful – set up his own business
- ♥ Similar education level and we have a few friends in common
- ♥ Fun
- ♥ Enthusiastic
- ♥ Makes me laugh
- ♥ Took me to a fantastic restaurant
- ♥ Makes me feel amazing when I'm with him
- ♥ Both of us share a sense of adventure to learn new things
- ♥ Great chemistry
- ♥ Kisses are amazing

Weaknesses

- ♠ I've been on two dates in the last month with him
- ♠ He takes a while to get back to me
- ♠ I slept with him on the second date and I'm feeling a little vulnerable now in case it was a two-date wonder
- ♠ He looks at himself in the mirror ten times more than I do
- ♠ He seems a bit showy
- ♠ He's always busy in work
- ♠ He's been late picking me up
- ♠ I seem to the one suggesting dating activities
- ♠ He doesn't talk about the future
- ♠ Negative dating pattern – he gives me crumbs

Opportunities

- ♥ I'll ask him if he is interested in signing up for a hike
- ♥ I won't text him for a week and see if he contacts me first
- ♥ I will invite him to a drinks afternoon that I'm having with friends next week

Threats

- ♠ Work will take over and be his only priority
- ♠ He's kind of showy with his possessions … is he just looking for another possession?
- ♠ Wasting my time on this guy means I will miss out on a guy who really does want a relationship

EXERCISE:
SWOT YOUR DATE

Strengths

Weaknesses

Opportunities

Threats

So what did you find? Do you play off each other's strengths and shore up each other's weaknesses? What opportunities do you have together? And perhaps most importantly, what are the threats to this relationship, and can they be addressed? For example, if you're getting the feeling after a few dates that he isn't looking for a relationship, call him on it. Say to him, 'Look, I think you're hot and I think we get along really well together, but I'm just checking in with you to see what you're looking for. If this isn't the right time, that's fine. I'd much rather know today than six months from now. I still think you're hot either way, though!' It's okay to call guys out – how else are you going to know? And remember, women are very intuitive, so trust this quality in yourself.

The Marketing Mix

If you were a tube of toothpaste or a bottle of shampoo, a marketing guru would take one look at you and decide exactly how to get you directly into the hands of consumers. Too bad you can't do the same for your love life. Or can you?

Taking a cue from the corporate world again, let's look at a few marketing principles to see how they can be applied to your search for love.

Follow the four Ps

When approaching a new project, marketers divide the task into manageable pieces: product, price, place and promotion. 'The four Ps' is a common business model used to market just about anything, so why not love?

1. Product

Your product is the core of your marketing effort. It must be something desirable. Look at it this way — if you have the best chocolate bar in the world but you're not packaging it right, it will never get bought. Fact. Of course it's what's inside that counts, but at the start it's all about the visuals. So make sure you have your product, i.e. *you*, packaged right before you go anywhere.

You must also understand what the buyer (in this case, men) is looking for. While every man is different, there are certain things about a woman that will make any man stand up, take notice and make him decide he wants to get to know her on a deeper level. We'll go into this in more detail later, but for now, suffice it to say that men are looking for a woman who is fun, attractive, sexy, emotionally stable, independent, high valued, feminine and open to adventure. By knowing what your market (men) wants, you can be more effective in dating. In other words, being a boring date just won't cut it.

Product testing is a key part of the first P, which in dating terminology means more dates! You aren't going to get this right on date one, but the more dates you go on, the more chances you have of delivering the best version of yourself to the dating marketplace.

2. Placement

You've got the right product. Now you need to know the right places to go to promote the fact that you are single and available. You wouldn't believe the amount of amazing, desirable, feminine, successful, well-packaged women who haven't been on a date in ages because they simply do not go out and meet men. In business, *place* is where the customer meets the salesperson, be it face to face in a shop, an office, a trade fair or online. Ladies, I know this is simple stuff, but where are you selling your product? Where is your point of sale for yourself?

3. Promotion

In business, promotion is how the market tells buyers about the product. When I do a client consultation, I often get people to write down the ideal person they want to be and then think about how that person would dress and act. Because packaging is so important, you must work out what you want to say with your clothes. Your choice of colour, style and shape will speak volumes about the person you are.

And like any desirable commodity, appearance is everything. You have to make yourself as attractive as possible everywhere you go. You can slice it any way you want, but men are visual, so you need to promote yourself the best way you can. If this means spending more time and money making yourself look good, well then, you just have to do it. Men absolutely judge books by their covers, so you need to make yours as spectacular and eye-catching as it can be. This goes for both your online dating personality and your real-life one.

4. Pricing

How much value do you put on yourself? When it comes to assessing your value and the type of person you aspire to have a relationship with, you need to be realistic. If you place too much value on yourself, men will never meet your expectations and you will come across as too much of a challenge. Yes, it's great that your self-esteem is sky high, but putting an inappropriate value on yourself and having unrealistic expectations may cost you time and missed opportunities if your bar is set too high. You may need to knock yourself off your own pedestal and set lower expectations. Look at things more realistically in terms of the men and the environment. You might want to marry a successful, good-looking millionaire, but there just might not be any in your area.

At the same time, it's also important not to undervalue yourself. I know this sounds like a complete contradiction, but only you can find the right balance for you. It sounds clichéd, but at the end of the day, you can lose weight, you can revamp your image and you can say all the right things during a conversation, but if you don't value yourself, then how can anyone value you back? If you want to meet a great guy, you have to be great yourself. You must lead a valuable life full of passionate activities that enrich you. If you are not living that life, how can you expect to attract a great guy who is? Cultivating a high-value life is the first step in attracting the love you deserve. Remember, your Mr Right is hoping to find a woman of high value too, not someone he has to fix.

The trick here is to find the balance of truly living (and not pretending to live) a high-value life and having realistic expectations of your partner. And let's face it – a woman with real value and integrity is not going to put up with a guy who doesn't have those qualities too.

You don't need business expertise to understand the four Ps. You only need to realise that just as products get market results every day, by adopting a marketing approach to your dating life, you will start meeting great guys and getting real results too.

Destructive Dating Patterns

Albert Einstein said, 'The definition of insanity is doing the same thing over and over again and expecting different results.' Doing the same thing time after time and expecting that it will turn out differently this time is a poor strategy for dating success too. For example, here are some excellent ways to make sure you will stay stuck:

- ♥ You keep going for the same player guys and accepting the same crumbs you've been thrown from every other guy.
- ♥ You keep wondering why you can't keep weight off when you've made no long-term changes to your diet and you never exercise.
- ♥ You're desperate to find someone but you stay in every weekend watching TV.
- ♥ You complain that there are no men out there, but at the same time you're not making sure that you feel and look great.
- ♥ You feel self-conscious or lack in self-esteem, but you're not looking for ways to make yourself feel better.

If you're stuck in a pattern that's not getting you what you want in your dating life, then it's time to change the pattern. And that means changing the only part of the situation you have control over – you.

Here are a few of the destructive patterns that I see most often.

1. The single victim mentality

What is holding back your dating life? You could blame your family, the logistics of it all, your job, your education, men, religion, your boss or your kids, but where are *you* in that list? Each of the people you mentioned has no idea that you are holding them responsible for your lame dating life. And I'm sorry to say it, but your age isn't a good excuse either. Yes, it will be more difficult to date as you get older since the dating pool is smaller, but singles are meeting older singles every day.

A woman who came to one of my singles events told me that it was my fault she wasn't having a good time and men weren't approaching her, even though she had sat in the corner with an awful puss on her face, did nothing to engage with any man and gave out about all the men who were there. So I suggested she look at where the words were coming from. You need to take responsibility for the stories you tell to others about your dating life and about yourself. It's nobody's fault that you're feeling the way you are.

Or to give you another example, a lot of women come to me and say there was no spark on the date. I simply ask them if they did anything to induce the spark, and nine times out of 10, the answer is no. They sat there the entire time waiting for a spark to hit them on the head. Instant chemistry can happen, but only for the lucky few. And even if it does happen, you have to be open to it.

Remember, nothing outside of you can make you feel anything – only you can control how you feel. You are the only one who can change your dating life. You must take full responsibility for your dating life up to now. You must be willing to change your perspective on love and be willing to do the hard work necessary, for however long it takes, to create personal change and transform your dating life.

EXERCISE:
SIGN ON THE DOTTED LINE

Here are some helpful affirmations for taking full self-responsibility. I want you to say them aloud and then sign on the dotted line.

- ♥ I am completely responsible for my dating life.
- ♥ I am completely responsible for all my own feelings and actions, and I decide what to do with them.
- ♥ I am completely responsible for my emotional and physical health.
- ♥ I give others complete responsibility for their feelings and actions. (You can't control how other people feel about you.)
- ♥ I take responsibility for expressing my true essence in the world in positive and loving ways.
- ♥ I take complete responsibility for doing the exercises and making and keeping the agreements set out in this book – no excuses!

Name: ....

Date: ....

2. Prince Charming

Unrealistic expectations can cause a lot of damage to your dating life and relationships. What little girl doesn't grow up listening to fairytales and hoping to be swept off her feet by a handsome, rich prince? These stories wedge themselves into our subconscious minds and create a paradigm for romantic relationships that sets us up for failure. There are plenty of examples in modern films: just think of *Pretty Woman* or *Cinderella*. This ultimately means that a lot of women would rather wait around to be saved than do anything about it themselves. Or worse still, they take on someone who is more like a Prince Harming than a Prince Charming. Sure, he may be sexy, smart, rich and funny, but he might also be a liar and a cheat.

If you are genuine about meeting someone for a relationship, you have to stay in reality and forget about the fairytales. Stop focusing on Prince Charming and start focusing on what type of relationship you want that fits in with your life plan. You need to do a daily and weekly reality check. The following questions might help you.

EXERCISE:
IS HE A FROG OR A PRINCE?

1. If you took away all the superficial stuff – the looks and the money – is this guy good for you?
2. Do you think this guy is interested in you or does he just want a quick grope?
3. Does he have a good character? Will he be a positive influence on you?

If the guy scores three for three, you're heading to Prince Charming territory.

3. I can fix him

We've all dated a few duds. Maybe it was the guy who couldn't hold down a job, the guy who was an obvious player or even the guy who, oops, forgot to tell you he had a wife or girlfriend. There's no problem having one date with these guys – they'll probably wine and dine you. But why do women continue to put up with their crap and think they will change?

Shut down the drama in your life. It's unhealthy. Arguing and fighting create dis-ease. Stay away from negative, selfish, energy-draining relationships that do not honour you, or even worse, use you, abuse you and take advantage of your kindness. Don't buy into his negativity or guilt trips. Don't try to change others – there's enough work to do on yourself. Develop relationships where you both can grow with mutual respect, love and appreciation.

Confession: a few years ago I dated a confident, dashing, 30-year-old solicitor. To be honest, I didn't even like him. I found him rude and obnoxious and I didn't like the way he spoke to wait staff when we were out. He was so arrogant and always belittled my job with snobby comments. I hate admitting this, but I put up with his abuse for about two months. I look back on it now in horror, but at the time I had major self-esteem issues and I felt that if I could fix him and make him like me, then everything else would be okay. He was like ice cream – I knew he was bad for me, but my self-esteem was so low at the time that I wanted to sabotage myself, only to feel 10 times worse afterwards.

Eventually, I told him where to go. I decided to work on my self-esteem for a while and enlisted in a confidence-building workshop before I dated anyone else.

If my story rings true with you, then you need to decide if you are ready to break the loser cycle. Here's how.

1. If you find yourself consistently dating unavailable men, whether they're married or simply emotionally unavailable, ask yourself why. You may lack confidence, you may have intimacy issues or you may simply not want commitment. If these things bother you, you can get help from a counsellor. Work on yourself for a while. To start, write down five things you like about yourself and ask your friends and family to tell you five things they like about you.

2. Ask yourself where you are meeting these losers and try to see if there is a pattern. For example, if you met your last three loser dates in the bar, then you need to find a new place to meet guys. I love bars, but unfortunately bars and clubs can be a nesting ground for players. Wherever it is, if you keep meeting losers in a particular place, you need to break the cycle.

3. What signals are you sending him? Sometimes it's not him, it's you. If all you want is a casual relationship, then you'll attract the guys who just want flings. There are plenty of single men who aren't interested in commitment either, so date them instead. On the opposite end of the spectrum, if this isn't for you, then don't feel that you have to play down your desire for a relationship just so you won't scare him away. If you want a relationship, say so! If he's only in it for a fling, you don't want him anyway, so stop wasting your time with him. Weed him out early on so that you're free to find the guy who *will* fit in with what you want.

4. Alpha females

I have many alpha females as clients who are very successful in business and in their careers, but they're coming up short in their dating lives and can't understand why. It drives them crazy, since they're able to control every other part of their lives. But that's the key word here: *control*. These women often come across as too controlling, and men think they'll be emasculated because they won't be allowed to be themselves and the woman will always be trying to take the reins away from them.

Let me tell you about one such client, Joanne, and how learning how to tap into her feminine power worked wonders for her.

Joanne is VP of Sales at a top international company. At 5'11, Joanne is tall and very attractive and she already has a strong physical presence. She's a powerhouse at work and she knows how to get the job done quickly and efficiently. She's a true alpha female and her approach at work has brought her great success.

The problem was that on every date I set her up on, she bamboozled the guys with her success stories and her presence. She controlled the date from the start, as she thought that she knew all the best restaurants in town and that he wouldn't pick a good one, and she insisted on going Dutch on the date. She wasn't able to flip off the alpha female switch outside of work, and it was sending men running to the hills as fast as they could go.

During our coaching session, we looked at her dating patterns and decided she needed to practise being more feminine and stop trying to control the outcome. The first challenge I set her was to say four simple words that she hadn't said in years: 'I need your help.' This plays into all the good stuff about a man. Just as it's in our nature to nurture, it's in his DNA to make you feel protected, happy and cared for. The challenge was to do this simple exercise four times a week wherever she could, even at work.

So when she was on her way out of the supermarket, laden down with bags, she simply said to the security man, 'I need your help.' When she was in a meeting with a potential new client, who also just so happened to be a hot guy, instead of operating in her usual bullish sales mode, she said, 'I need your help.' When she was at the petrol pumps and saw a man she liked, she started the conversation with 'I need your help – do you know the best way to the city centre?' (Even though she had a satnav in her car.) And finally, when I set her up on a date and they were talking about their shared love of running, she said, 'I need your help in learning more about the nutrition side of things.' They spent the next hour talking about it, and her date shared a lot about why nutrition is so important to him and how it has impacted his life, which was basically his way of trying to impress her. By the end of the conversation, he said that he'd send her a nutritional plan that he uses that would help her too.

Before Joanne started working with me, she only knew how to show her alpha side and it was turning men off. But then she saw that when she flipped the switch to her more feminine side, men were stepping over themselves to help her. Think Scarlett O'Hara in *Gone with the Wind*, sitting under the tree making every man feel understood and special as they begged to fetch food for her. You can have this, too.

It's worth mentioning that Joanne also made a decision to wear softer, more feminine clothing on her date versus her usual black suit that she wore straight from the office, which says alpha female loud and clear. If you have to wear a black suit to work, dress it up with a feminine coloured top inside, some nice jewellery or playful lipstick.

When you use your feminine side, men will feel like you really get them. They'll want to connect with you on that emotional level they crave with a woman. This is the power of the feminine mystique. Watch Joanie on *Mad Men* or Julia Roberts in *Pretty Woman* for examples of strong women who get their way by using their femininity and allowing men to help. (Remember the scene in *Pretty Woman* where the shop girls are mean to her and Richard Gere comes to her rescue, flashing his credit card? He ended up taking a whole day off work to help her.)

If you're in a relationship or dating when a man starts doing things for you, be gracious and thank him immediately. Let him know how much you appreciate what he's done for you, even if it's not the way you wanted it done. In many ways, men are like puppies: the more love, appreciation and respect they get from you, the more they will want to give and do for you. So like Joanne, I want you to try out your feminine wiles on men – male friends, business associates, strangers, dates, potential dates and/or your lovers – and watch how your life with men begins to change.

Here are some feminine qualities to embrace on a daily basis. Think about each quality and write down what you could do to bring more of this quality into your life. For example, think about a time when you were playful and then think about how you could bring some of that playfulness into your day today. The more you make a habit of embracing your feminine qualities, the more it will become part of your daily life naturally.

EXERCISE: EMBRACE YOUR FEMININE QUALITIES

Think about each quality and write down what you could do to bring more of this quality into your life. Feel free to add more qualities to this list.

1. Nurturing
2. Playful
3. Open
4. Sexy
5. Soft
6. Patient
7. Intuitive
8. Gentle
9. Sweet
10. Loving
11. Affectionate
12. Tactile
13. Empathetic
14. Receptive
15. Surrendering
16. Strong
17. Wise
18. Unselfish
19. Caring
20. Empowered
21. Sensual

5. The romance adrenaline junkie

My name is Avril and I'm a recovering romance adrenaline junkie. My dating history is chequered with plenty of short relationships that usually peaked at about three months. I guess you could say I was addicted to the high of early romance – the passion, the chemistry, the sex. I was also guilty of jumping into relationships head first and not really 'pre-qualifying' the men I dated past that initial attraction. This once nearly led me to board a boat to sail the Greek Isles on my own with a Frenchman who spoke limited English whom I had only met the night before. If it wasn't for my friend Orla, who lit it rip, God knows where I'd be now.

Why can rushing into a relationship lead to failure?

You're being too impulsive

When you lead with your heart and physical attraction, you can be blind to red flags. It's important to use your gut and attraction as gauges in choosing a mate, but they shouldn't be the only qualifiers in a relationship. If you have a tendency to be impulsive, make sure your calendar is booked up with other dates or work commitments or meet-ups with friends. By not giving yourself time to be impulsive, you will give yourself some breathing space to look at your date rationally.

You're forgetting to do a reality check

When you know what it is that you absolutely must have and must not have in a relationship, you can quickly pre-qualify whether or not someone is a good match. Take a deep breath and **SWOT** your man over and over again (see pages 55–59). It will save you a lot of heartache. Think about the precious time you are giving up if you go on a date with this guy. What else could you be doing? Is he really worth it? Could you be spending that time forging a relationship with someone more compatible?

You're getting physical too quickly

Sex is blooming amazing, but it can make you stupid. It can cloud your ability to judge a person's character, especially when the chemistry is off the charts. Sex is your decision and I'm not here to judge you on it, but if you want to be in a real, long-term and committed relationship, having sex too soon sends the wrong signal.

Take your time before you jump into bed with a guy. Having sex too soon and hoping it will lead to commitment is just trading short-term urges for long-term desires. So keep yourself out of the firing zone. Don't go back to a guy's house for the first few weeks and don't invite him back to yours. Remember, if a guy asks you back for tea, it doesn't mean tea. Usually he doesn't even have milk. And always remember that sex is not leverage for a relationship and that you are not the exception to the rule.

It's all about the BOOM!

If the chemistry is a 10+, you are in trouble. Like I said before, lots of clients come to me and say great guy, but no chemistry. On the other hand, I have a lot of clients who come to me and say the chemistry was out of this world even after the first date – it was boom, bang and fireworks. To be honest, I'm more concerned about the latter, as too much chemistry can make a girl boom herself right out of the ballpark.

A lot of men know exactly how to create chemistry with a woman. There are pick-up artist schools all over the world now, where nerdy, needy and greedy men learn how to pick up women. Be careful here. Keep yourself busy and don't allow the boom to control you – *you* control the boom. Take your time to forge a healthy relationship. It will be worth the wait.

6. Catch me if you can

The 'catch me if you can' type is all about fear. When you start to fall for someone, you end up pushing them away in case you get hurt. You set him up to fail so that you can control the heartbreak. At this stage, a diva can raise her ugly head. She will look for any excuse. It could be something simple, like him being a half hour late or if you thought he wasn't giving you enough attention. You will just end up sabotaging the relationship.

Kate met Anthony at a friend's BBQ and they immediately hit it off. Kate, 28, was a fun PR executive and Anthony, 33, was a nurse. They had so much in common and they both shared a sense of adventure for travel. Anthony had been engaged three years previously and was looking for a relationship. Kate loved to buzz around dating loads of men, but she had admitted to me that she really wanted a relationship and was actually quite lonely. Kate usually went for successful, charismatic types who often treated her like crap.

Anthony really liked Kate and after the BBQ he texted her to go on a date three days later. Anthony organised everything. He had heard that she liked the circus, so he found out about a quirky theatrical circus that was in town. Kate couldn't believe that someone could be so thoughtful. She was used to guys who just used her. Kate started having trouble sleeping and started to have commitment fears: *Why is he doing all of this? I'm not ready for this. He's coming across as a little needy.*

After the third date, Kate started being very sharp with Anthony and taking him up on his opinions. She stopped texting him back and started to become a little distant. Anthony persisted and invited her on a fourth date to meet his friends. Kate really wanted to go but said no, hoping that Anthony would call her and beg her to come out. He didn't, but later she texted him to say that she was in the area and she would pop in. Anthony was a little taken aback when she arrived and he picked up that there was a problem, so he introduced her to a few like-minded people and tried to give her space.

Kate really liked Anthony, but she was so afraid of someone actually treating her well. In the end, she wound up having a blow-out with Anthony in front of his friends over nothing. She stormed out of the bar, but on the bus home she realised what she was after doing. Meanwhile, though, Anthony was completely shocked and was left wondering who this person was and where the gorgeous, bubbly girl he had met a few weeks ago had gone.

Kate called Anthony the next day to explain, but unsurprisingly, he politely said he didn't want to see her again.

Kate is an extreme example of self-sabotage. She liked him, she didn't like him, she liked him, she didn't like him. The more interest Anthony showed in her, the more fear it instilled in Kate, to the point where she became a blubbering mess and orchestrated a gateway to get out. But the thing is, she really did like him.

Other people are not as dramatic as Kate and enjoy more fun on the run. They are happy and positive and live a seemingly wonderful life. They send flowery emails, make frequent phone calls and have fabulous first dates, but the grass is always greener somewhere else and they won't give anyone a chance. These people are just as fearful, as they don't really know what they are looking for and they tend to float from one date to the next. They fill themselves with so much fun and so many activities that they don't really have to think about their own lives.

Underlying our fears is a lack of trust in ourselves. It's okay to be afraid of relationships or indeed happiness, but when we don't acknowledge this fear, it will be transferred into a bodily symptom, anger or something equally destructive. So give these guys a chance. What's the worst that can happen?

7. The friends zone

You've got loads of best male friends. You cook dinners together, rent movies, crash in each other's apartments and for all intents and purposes you act like a couple. Maybe you have a crush on this guy but are afraid to ruin the friendship by getting romantically involved.

Claire ran her own business and came to me for dating coaching because she was struggling to meet men. She wore jeans and an oversized T-shirt but had an attractive face and a great figure. We set about creating her dating plan, but what struck me about Claire was how many men were already in her life. She was surrounded by them! She worked in a male-oriented environment, almost all her friends were men and she found it easy to chat and engage with men, but in her own words they were all 'just good friends' and at age 31 she hadn't had a long-term boyfriend in years. Claire met up with her 'boyfriends' every week for cinema nights and sports events and even invited them over for dinner, where they talked about their love lives. She had fancied a couple of the guys in the past, especially one guy in particular, John, but she didn't want to ruin the friendship and so she avoided meeting him for a while until her feelings subsided. John is now in a relationship.

Before going any further, let's define the 'friends zone', because understanding the problem can help you find the solution. Basically, the friends zone is where both individuals' needs are not getting met and there is a mismatch in romantic feelings. For example, there may be a sexual mismatch. You may not be sexually attracted to each other or have blocked out sexual feelings in order to stay safe in the friends zone. On the flip side, there may be a commitment mismatch, where only one person wants a relationship.

In any case, if you are genuinely looking for a relationship, friends zone relationships are wasted opportunities if you're not being fully satisfied. In a nutshell, by staying stuck in a friends zone relationship, you're not getting what you truly want and you're wasting your time.

EXERCISE:
10 MALE FRIENDS

Make a list of 10 male friends in your life. (If you don't have 10 male friends, that's no problem – just write down as many as you can think of) and categorise them as being a potential date for you. Guys can often slip into the friends zone without meaning to and they might be begging to get out.

1. ....
2. ....
3. ....
4. ....
5. ....
6. ....
7. ....
8. ....
9. ....
10. ....

♥ ♥ ♥

If there is someone on the list who you get on really well with but they can't give you the relationship that you need, keep him as a friend but don't expect anything else. On the other hand, if you think he has romantic feelings for you and that you are only stringing him along, then be direct with him. Otherwise it's unfair and you're wasting his time.

If you think there is someone on your list who could be a potential, then what's stopping you from finding out? Follow these tips.

Understand the different levels of love

My clinical hat is coming out here. Remember that love is a process. You don't just hop on a big fluffy cloud to Loveland. It's also not just a feeling. You don't suddenly wake up in the morning and say you love someone, like the same way that you might say you're feeling hungry.

There are several components to creating love, not just one single feeling. Love is a process as well as the feelings and emotions that go along with that process. The actual process unfolds in four stages:

1. Attraction
2. Connection
3. Intimacy
4. Commitment

The first stage is mainly physical attraction and is triggered by non-verbal signals we give through a combination of attitude, physique and clothing – our overall appearance. The next three stages are mainly about mental and emotional attraction – building rapport, making the connection easy and comfortable, creating intimacy (both emotional and sexual) and finally, shifting into commitment.

One of the reasons people end up being 'just friends' is that they are simply not attractive to the person they desire. They only create feelings of connection around them (like a good friend) without any attraction or seduction feelings. For any number of reasons, then, the 'friends zone' individual just doesn't have that spark to make the other person desire them, lust after them and want them in return.

Fortunately, you can learn to be more attractive physically. You can groom yourself better, wear sexier clothes, improve your body language, get in better shape and flirt better so that your friend can start to see you as a potential too. Because guess what? More often than not, it all begins with flirting.

Understand the different levels of flirting

We will go into more detail about flirting later, but for now I just want you to know that there are three different layers of flirting: public, social and private flirting.

- ♥ **Public flirting** is usually a fun and harmless interaction with another person. There are many situations where you probably don't even realise you're flirting. You banter with the guard on the street or share a joke with the barman on a night out. You smile and make chit chat with your barista when you pick up your morning coffee. You give out about the weather to your taxi man. Public flirting happens all around us. But after a while, you will decide that a particular flirting connection will warrant a more individual focus, and then you'll need to move up a gear to social flirting.

- ♥ **Social flirting** is about making a personal connection, initiating chemistry and allowing your sexuality to ignite. It adds a promise–withdraw element to the mix by signalling interest, kind of like 'catch me if you can and see what might happen'. A woman can lick her lips, play with her hair, use sexually charged words, run her hand down her thigh, 'accidentally' brush up against someone or simply make eye contact with them.

- ♥ **Private flirting** is about two people uncovering and responding to each other's energy. It exudes sexual energy and intensifies playfulness. Understanding the difference between cute and sexy is what differentiates the men from the boys and the women from the girls.

Stop being so nice

Another reason why people end up in the friends zone is that they are too afraid, uncertain, passive or just too nice. Many people approach someone they are attracted to as 'just a friend' because it's less emotionally risky, so they pick the easier option. Being too nice and not stepping out of line is one of the most useless pieces of advice that was drilled into us when we were in school. It stops us from communicating and doing what we want. Be bold, face the fear and do it anyway. Ask the guy on a proper date, complete with romantic candles and a chemistry-inducing atmosphere, get outside of your comfort zone and flirt. If he cancels the date or isn't interested in your advances, then it's better to simply walk away and find someone who is.

If you're looking for a relationship, stop putting your time and energy into friends who aren't giving you what you need. You deserve to have what you want, so don't settle for a 'friends zone' situation that makes you miserable. Find someone who will be good enough to give you what you need.

8. Picky pandemic

Are you being too picky? One of my pet hates in my industry is the picky pandemic. Some people think that I'm actually a modelmaker, not a matchmaker. They have impossible-to-meet standards and they wear their massive checklists on their sleeves. Both men and women are responsible for this pandemic. Women, you know who are, and I can see you coming a mile away. They are usually the types whose eye shadow matches their toenails. Everything is in control and perfect in their lives, even though they're still, well, inexplicably single.

Take **Susan**, 37, an attractive, privately schooled accountant who comes from a privileged part of town. Susan came to me after trying two different introduction agencies. She had spent a lot of money trying to find her type, but to no avail. Susan still lived in the same area she'd grown up in. Her best friends from school were still her best friends.

They'd all gone to the same university and had followed similar career paths, married similar guys and went on similar holidays. They even liked similar fashion trends. Susan liked nothing more than meeting up with the girls and heading to the top designer shops followed by a glass of vino in their favourite hotspot in town.

However, this was happening less and less often as most of her girlfriends were married and babies were now the main topic of conversation. Susan was beginning to feel like the odd one out as she didn't have the 'man' part. She had attended all her friends' weddings but was wondering when her time would come. She was searching for a guy who was similar to her friends' guys, but better. He had to be a successful businessman, over six feet tall with a toned physique who had also attended a private school, drove a big car, preferably an Audi A6, liked rugby (since that's what all her friends' husbands did, so they could all go to rugby matches together) and was from an equally privileged area in town – preferably from the same area, actually – who could be slotted into her life and they would all live happily ever after. Over the past six months, Susan had spent a considerable amount of money trying to find Mr Perfect, but none of them got past the first date. Some of them didn't even get past the initial phone call because their voice didn't fit her ideal.

Does this sound even a little bit like you?

Look, ladies, I've worked in this industry for a long time and I understand the environment. I'm honest with all my clients. I want to meet their expectations and I genuinely want to get as many things as I can right on their application form. But oftentimes this type of client would be better off just ripping up their application form and throwing it in the bin, as it's completely unrealistic and often just plain shallow.

Do you think you have a case of the picky pandemic? Or do you never give anyone a chance to invest in you? Do you believe there is one guy out there for you? If so, how do you manage your expectations without selling yourself short?

There's a difference between being picky and being unrealistic. But first, a disclaimer: at some level, you *should* be picky. After all, if your goal is marriage, we're talking about the one person you're going to spend the rest of your life with, so being a little choosy goes a long way. It's arguable that plenty of people aren't picky *enough*.

Bottom line? People are looking for the wrong things. You should have high standards, but people are too picky about the things that aren't important – and not picky enough about the things that are.

So how do you determine what is truly important and what isn't? Many people are willing to concede – or at least they know that they *should* concede – that looks are really only skin deep. Yet they still explicitly rule out, for example, short men, bald men or even men who have a weird walk. They say things like, 'That's just not what I'm attracted to.' I can tell you now that one of the most important things I learned from my 40 dates in 40 days experience is that you should never, ever judge a book by its cover. Several times I was attracted to a guy who initially I wouldn't have thought I'd be visually attracted to whatsoever, but I let myself be open to other parts of his character and realised that he had other very appealing attributes.

And here's a shocker – attraction isn't the most important thing. That doesn't mean you need to give up on lust, passion or even simple chemistry. It just means that it might not hit you like a lightning bolt when you walk into the first date saloon and that you should at least give it a chance to develop, even with people you might not consider to be your type. Why? Because then you can focus on what *is* important. Not the person 'on paper' or in a vacuum, but on the relationship (whatever that is, either casual or long term) you can potentially build with someone.

If your parents, or even your grandparents, are still together, ask them their secret. I'm willing to bet that they won't say that they are still together because they think the other person is smoking hot. It's the 'boring' stuff – the trust, laughter, honesty, compassion and shared values – that they will talk about. That's the stuff that can only partially reveal itself on date one but is your job to find out. So try not to be so clouded by visual chemistry and to look at what's going to endure after the initial thrill is gone, because hasty rejections can lead to missed opportunities.

If you need some too-picky therapy, just think of it this way: you're not lowering your standards, you're expanding them. Here's how: edit your checklist. You are only allowed three essential requirements and none of them can be phys-ical attributes. For example, it could be something like 'kind to others, intellectually curious, likes animals', or if you're not into pets, 'wants children' (as far as you can tell on date #1). Go on a second date – anyone who passes your three-point checklist gets to date #2, and I mean anyone.

Broaden your type, but trust your gut. If after two dates you honestly can't see it working out – if you struggle to make conversation or you clash on a moral principle – you can let it go guilt free. After all, you've got to make time for all the new possibilities you've now opened up for yourself.

Colette, an intelligent, attractive, loving woman, fell in love when she was 23 with a charming, charismatic, handsome man she met in college. She was married at 27 but the marriage ended after five years when she found out he had a wandering eye and had got off with her best friend before the wedding. After her failed marriage, she fell head over heels in love with a guy who was a carbon copy of her ex-husband. It was full of passion, lust and chemistry, but it only lasted for six months because he didn't want to commit to anything long term and he wanted to concentrate on his growing business.

It took her a long time to get over the subsequent (and predictable) heartbreak. Colette started to question the meaning of love and relationships and her own judgement. From what I learned about Colette and her relationships, it seemed clear that both times she ignored selfish, egocentric and bullish tendencies because of what came with the rest of the package – someone who was also handsome, charming and passionate.

Colette decided to break the mould because she wanted a true partner and she wanted to evolve past her destructive dating patterns. I encouraged Colette to date several different kinds of men for the first time in her life, as she had missed out on the dating scene in her twenties. We also discussed how to manage her tendency to be swept away by chemistry and how to see other attributes in men.

This is what Collette wrote to me: 'I just want to say thank you. After a mere nine months after starting the process, I am with a man who is crazy about me and within a short space of time we have already talked about the future. It's funny, he knew very quickly that he wanted to be exclusive and wanted to share it with me. He's a man of integrity and character; a man who I'm attracted to and have great sex with; he's a man who really wants to know me; a man who cheers me on in every part of my life; a man who introduced me to his family and friends from the get go; a man who loves my family and they love him; a man who integrates me into his life and loves being part of mine; a man who said "I love you" first; and a man who says, "I want to help you make your dreams come true."

'The extreme chemistry wasn't there at the start and being honest is still not there now compared to before. I don't get giddy or sick to my stomach around him. For a while that confused me because that's what I thought love was. But now I just know, for the first time ever, that I'm with a real partner who is going to be there for me every day – who has eyes only for me and is genuinely interested in me and our relationship.

'Thank you, Avril, for helping me to make a conscious effort to break my cycle and get me back out there. It worked.'

EXERCISE:
YOUR DATING LIFE

Think about your dating life – the guys you have dated, wanted to date or past relationships. Now answer the following questions.

1. Which of the above dating patterns feels the closest to your own?

_____

2. Is this pattern compatible with your dating goals?

_____

3. Are there any similarities between the guys you have dated?

4. If these relationships ended poorly, are there any similarities?

5. Could you have done something differently? For example, did your boyfriend say you were too controlling or that you talked about yourself too much? Did you argue a lot? Did you get off with someone else?

6. Do you only date attractive and successful men? If yes, why?

7. Do you think that you date certain types for a reason?

8. Do you believe in love at first sight?

9. Do you tend to chase guys?

10. Do you think there is something that you could do to make sure your relationships work better in the future?

♥ ♥ ♥

If you answered 'yes' to more than three of these questions, then you need to decide right now to do something different, as your strategy is definitely not working. Change your behaviour and take a new approach to your dating life. When you act differently, like flirting or deciding to not always be the nice girl, other people have something new to react to. The result might not be the perfect outcome and you might not meet your Prince Charming, but it will be something different, offering new possibilities and less heartache.

EXERCISE: DO SOMETHING DIFFERENT

What pattern(s) have you decided will not be part of your life anymore?

....

....

What are you going to differently?

....

....

When will you know that you are not in the same pattern any more?

....

....

❤ ❤ ❤

Break the destructive cycle

You might think you couldn't possibly be hindering your own dating success. It's a lot easier to blame the environment, blame men, give in to the single victim mentality or believe the fairytales. But you are a bigger factor in this equation than you think. You can't control a man's opinion or how he acts towards you, but you can control your response.

If you're honest about your dating patterns, you may find a few common problems that are sabotaging any potential relationship. At some point, you have to identify what's going wrong. Maybe it's the men you choose. Maybe it's your addiction to fantasy or maybe it's because you are simply not trying at all. Be strong and deal with what might be holding you back from the relationship you want. It's difficult to break destructive patterns. You might get frustrated and think it's too hard to change. It may take time and you may find yourself slipping back into your old habits again. But the sooner you address these destructive patterns, the sooner you will feel better about yourself and the closer you will be to meeting the right man.

Mr Wrong

One of the most common things I hear about in the media is that everyone is looking for Mr Right. But let's look at Mr Wrong for a minute.

As a matchmaker, I'm constantly working with clients to refine their choices. When I ask them to tell me what they want, they fire off a ream of attributes like they're ordering from a takeaway. But when I ask them what they definitely *don't* want, that part of the form is often left blank.

Accentuate the positive

I know there have probably been times in your past when you thought you'd met the right man and yet he turned out, like all the others, to be wrong. I want you to make sure you don't waste time on the wrong men and instead learn to invest in the good ones. It's not easy and it doesn't always come naturally, but it has some incredible rewards.

Which is why I'm going to give you a list of three essentials. Over the next few months, I want you to go on third dates and beyond with guys who:

1. Prioritise you
2. Accept you
3. Are consistent with you

I'll always remember when my good friend **Áine** started seeing Alfie, whom she met through their shared love of horses. He'd been chasing her for ages but she never gave him the time of day. Eventually she gave him a shot and went on a date with him, but she wasn't all that keen on him. She told me he was a bit rough around the edges – a farmer who wouldn't fit into her busy city social life, didn't dress the way she liked and was so uninhibited that he was liable to say anything. He persisted, though, and kept asking her out.

Áine had been seeing Alfie for about four weeks when she was involved in a very bad equestrian accident. She was in hospital for months and at first she was told she'd never walk again. Her family remained at her bedside every day … and so did Alfie. He drove two hours every day, over and back from his farm, just to be with her. Some days she was angry, some days she was depressed, some days she was sick, but he never missed a day. Thankfully, after intense rehabilitation, Áine has made a 90% recovery. She will never ride horses again, she has lost part of the strength in her legs and she had to give up her top corporate job in the city. However, she gained the knowledge that Alfie loved her eternally, whether she walked or not.

Three months after Áine was discharged from the hospital, she moved in with Alfie. Áine and Alfie now have a beautiful baby daughter.

Thankfully we don't all have such extreme experiences as Áine's that make us re-evaluate our life and our priorities. But think about this – if you stripped away your looks, your home, your career and your money, you'd only be left with everything that's on the *inside*. You'd be left with your kindness, your generosity, your sense of humour. You'd be left with your mind, your heart, your spirit.

So if you've struggled to figure out why you choose the wrong men, the answer is right there in front of you: you've been investing in the least important qualities. Looks come and go. Jobs come and go. Money comes and goes. I know this may sound nicey-nicey airy-fairy, but I believe this is one of the biggest things that holds women back in a relationship. They are so hell bent on the perfect traits that they forget the basics.

There is no shortage of impressive men out there who make you tingle every time you think about them, but they're worthless if they don't put *you* first. You need to stop chasing these men and getting sucked in by their charm, their wit, their looks or their money.

Instead, look for a guy who does what he says, who says what he means and who makes it clear that you're a priority to him, then learn to appreciate these fundamental traits even more. After all, the guy who doesn't prioritise you now is never going to.

Eliminate the negative

You need to be clear about what you're looking for. You need to know your negotiables and your non-negotiables. You need to be specific but you also need to be open to whatever presents itself. The busier you are in your dating life, the more chances you will have of meeting a man you will connect with. But if a guy doesn't fit, move on.

You also need to understand that you can't change someone. Ever. If a guy isn't a passionate man, you can't turn him into one who is. If he isn't interested in family, you can't make him want to have kids. If he's negative, you're not going to turn him into a positive, reflective person unless you want to be his therapist.

You need to find someone who is ready and shares the same mindset as you. Here are a few pitfalls to watch out for.

Timing is everything

You aren't going to turn a guy who's looking for a fling into a marriage-minded man, and if you're seeing a married man, don't expect him to leave his wife for you. It's just not the right time for him, so don't blame him and don't try to change him. Perhaps your paths will cross again six months from now and you both will be looking for a relationship then. Timing is everything.

Money can't buy you love

A lot of women want me to find them someone rich and successful. But beware of the big spenders. Oftentimes you are no different to the flashy car they drive or the expensive watch on their wrist – they will treat you like just another one of their possessions or will see you as a trophy wife. Just because a guy has a big bank balance doesn't mean he will adore you in the way that you deserve to be adored.

Jason, 34, came into my office last year for a matchmaking consultation. He had read about me in a newspaper and thought I could help him. He was very attractive, very confident and very successful.

Part of my consultation requires filling out an application form beforehand, but he didn't do it and said he didn't have the time. That should have set the alarm bells ringing, but against my better judgement, I took him on as a client. He made it quite clear that money was no object. He even sent me a massive bouquet of roses at my office. I wasn't sure if he was interested in me or if he was just showing off.

I set him up on a date with Kathy, an attractive, intelligent, fun girl who worked in PR and was a complete treasure. It was obvious that they were a great match and I was sure there would be a second date. I patted myself on the back for a job well done.

However, Kathy rang a month later to ask to be put back on my books. The second date never happened. He kept cancelling, saying something in work came up that he just had to sort out, or that he was really tired after a long week, or that he was heading away with the lads on a boys' weekend, or, or, or.

Ironically, I bumped into Jason that weekend out on the town. He was on a date with a super hot, super skinny 20-year-old who was done up like a doll and was gloating about what amazing restaurant he had just brought her to.

What Jason was saying and doing were two completely different things. There was no point working with a client like this, so I told him I was freezing his membership. His mindset was all wrong and nobody could change that, only himself.

If you really want to be with someone who is successful, look for someone who is passionate and primed for success. You want someone who is passionate about life, their work and what they do, their interests, their friends – and passionate about you.

He's looking for Ms Perfect

Beware of the guy who's never been in a relationship. Sorry to be a little stereotypical here, but these are often successful men in their mid-forties who have never married. Many of these men are looking for perfection.

You'll need to find out more about this guy on the first date. Why is he single? If he reels off a long list of attributes that he is looking for a woman, run quick, as you will never measure up.

Don't discount the divorcees

On the flip side of the coin, sometimes there's a good reason why a man is single later in life. Maybe he worked really hard in his twenties or he lived with a woman for a few years and got his heart broken. Don't be too quick to judge on a first date if he tells you that he has had loads of relationships or was married before.

Some women who come to me won't even contemplate meeting a man who was married before or has kids from another relationship. But meeting someone with no baggage whatsoever is unrealistic. If he has kids from a previous relationship, ask questions to try to suss out what kind of father he is. How does he manage that situation? How often does he see his kids? If his kids aren't talking to him, alarm bells should ring.

Don't discount all the wonderful guys who are divorced. He got married, he admitted the mistake and he moved on. As long as the relationship ended amicably (or as amicably as can be) and he learned from the experience, he's someone worth going for.

I will always remember **Kevin**, 41, coming into my office. He arrived bang on time with his application perfectly filled out. He was unassuming and shy, the kind of guy who was attractive but didn't know it. I later found out that Kevin had owned two top companies in the environment field, had an MBA from Harvard, had written several books and was now going back to university to study medicine. Kevin was genuine in his manner and was passionate about making a difference, yet he never bragged about his achievements. You would never find Kevin falling around the Dublin pubs either – he tended to prefer mini-breaks, reading and running.

Kevin married when he was 35, but the marriage ended after only nine months. He found the whole ordeal very difficult, as he genuinely wanted the marriage to work, but he said they hadn't been a good match from the start and he soon realised that she was the wrong one. Kevin came to me to help him find the right one. He never said anything negative about his ex-wife. He realised that family was really important to him. Why should a guy like him be punished for a mistake? He was ready to start again. I introduced him to Anna, a down-to-earth, fun and creative 37-year-old. They are still dating.

However, you do need to be careful with guys who want to make up for all their past mistakes. Or if he talks about his wife like she's the nastiest bitch from hell or he ran off with a 20-year-old, you might have a man who's just plain angry on your hands.

You can't fix him

I know a woman who first saw her husband at a funeral and thought he looked sad, so she spent her whole life trying to fix him and make him happy. You aren't looking for a guy to fix. You want a guy who has dealt with his crap and who can add to your life and you to theirs.

You want someone with the same mindset and timing as you. You may have different passions in life and that's fine, but you can't change someone's core characteristics. So when you're on a date, listen very carefully to figure out what his core characteristics and values are and trust your gut. If it feels wrong, it probably is.

He's not the one

It can be so confusing when you meet a great man and have an instant connection but he doesn't make any moves to get closer or commit to you.

If you're wondering what's going on and what he'll do next instead of just enjoying his attention and affection, you're in good company – it happens to so many of us. We attach ourselves to a man and invest our time and hearts in him, yet he feels slightly beyond our reach. And because we're so attached, we start making excuses for him when he's not showering us with the attention we crave.

I used to be so forgiving of the men I was dating, even though it hurt me. I brought one man to a birthday party where he was meeting my friends for the first time, but he spent the entire night talking to an old girlfriend who was there. It was humiliating. But I kept seeing him even though I knew he wasn't really committing to me. I'm telling you this embarrassing story so that you won't accept any kind of behaviour that doesn't feel good to you. If you let people mistreat you, they will.

When we get so focused on any one man, it's easy to be blinded. But try to remember that the end goal is a *relationship*, not him. It's like a game – the prize is the trophy, not the competing team. This might sound simple enough, but most of us do just the opposite and get sucked into the man, not the prize. No man is the prize. You should never feel like he's your man of choice or that you are his without a commitment from him.

So what do you say to a guy you've had a couple of dates with and who has potential if he asks you what you're looking for? Well, the man should never feel any kind of eagerness or neediness from you or feel like he is a prize of any kind. Keep to the facts of your plan and tell him truthfully where you're at. That way, you are being true to yourself without putting pressure on him. You could say something like this: 'Well, I don't want a serious boyfriend. I'm looking for a great guy to share a sexy, fun and amazing relationship with. And I don't want to get exclusive with anyone until that guy shows up.'

And that's it. You don't need to ask him anything and you don't need to discuss it anymore. Stick to the facts and you'll be calm, cool and collected. You should also keep dating other men until you get the kind of commitment that makes you happy.

I know this is hard, but trust me when I say that by doing this, you are doing the best thing you possibly can to ensure your happiness. No man should ever feel like he's your man of choice, he's your 'one' or that you're only seeing him – not until he's committed.

♥

Breaking Up Is Hard to Do

Hi Avril,

My boyfriend of five years broke up with me three months ago and I'm still devastated. We are both in our thirties, so we're not kids. To be honest, I don't know what happened. I thought it was all going great! He just told me that he couldn't imagine having a future with me. But the thing is, I did! My whole life was planned out with him in it. I've had to move back into my parents' house and I just feel so worthless. The strange thing is that he is still texting me and last week he told me he still has our picture in his phone and he really misses me. I've begged him to meet me and we did and we ended up in bed together. I thought that we would get back together, but the next morning he still insisted that he did not want to be with me. I can't get the whole thing out of my mind. I'm so confused. My friends are telling me that I need to get out, but I can't bear to be back single again. In any case, I will never meet anyone like him again. Please help!

Louise, Dublin

Louise, there is no easy way to say this: break-ups are crap! You need time to heal and even grieve. You sound like you loved your ex. You sound like you really miss your ex. You sound like you feel uncertain about your future. But if you stay stuck on your ex – if you stay stuck in the past or if you keep waiting for him to come back to you – you are depriving yourself of the chance to find someone who really loves you.

Louise, you said that it was all going great and that you don't know what happened. Is that really the case? You really didn't see any cracks? I want you to be honest with yourself. Do you really want to spend the rest of your life with someone who doesn't love you? Do you really want to spend the rest of your days with a man who throws you a few crumbs just to get you into bed, even though he knows that you want more and that you will feel even worse afterwards? I'm sorry, but I see him as egotistical and selfish. He is only thinking of his own needs. Do you really want to be in a relationship with a man like that?

You see, you have decided to only look at all the good attributes about your ex, but what you really need to do is crank up the bad memories so that you'll want to get over him as quickly as possible. In the same way that you fell in love with your ex, you need to learn how to fall out of love with him.

I want you to write down all the times your ex treated you badly, all the times he let you down and all the times he made you feel bad. Make the list as long or as short as you want, but really concentrate on each memory and really feel every negative feeling associated with that memory of him treating you badly. Now make it big and life-sized, so that you are actually in the memory. Keep replaying each memory until you are ultimately sick to your stomach, until you find yourself getting really angry and feeling that you just can't take it anymore.

Now imagine yourself looking at him and walking out the door and never having to feel those feelings again. Imagine yourself slamming the door behind you, and keep on walking. While you walk, imagine yourself feeling happy, fabulous and free. Feel all the excitement building up inside you as you step onto the new path of your positive, fun and loving future.

Louise, every time you start to miss your ex, I want you to do the above exercise until you fall in love with your new, exciting life again. The more you do it, the closer you will come to getting over the relationship and moving on.

Break-ups are hard, but a lot of singles make it worse by staying stuck for days, weeks, months or maybe even years. Basically, Louise is right – she won't meet anyone like her ex again. But the thing is, would she really want to? If you don't put your ex in the past, how can you put somebody else into your future?

Ending a relationship is never easy. It's going to leave a wound, but I promise that you'll eventually heal.

EXERCISE:
RAMP UP THE NEGATIVES

If you're going through a recent break-up where he broke up with you, then do the above exercise, ramping up the negatives and the reasons you broke up. State three negative things or weaknesses about him and begin.

1. ....

2. ....

3. ....

You need to get to the point of saying to yourself and your friends and family that it's *over*. But you can't just say it — you have to mean it. You must also break your own emotional bond and attachment to him. This is so important, but it's where a lot of women fail. They keep holding onto a fantasy emotional attachment for months or even years without him ever knowing. You must cut these emotional attachments once and for all or you will never move on. Don't be ambiguous. I can't stress this enough.

Too many women don't want to admit to themselves that it's over, so they try to soften the blow by saying things like, 'Things aren't working out right now, but that doesn't mean he'll always feel that way.' If you leave the door open even just a little bit, you walk away thinking you've still got a chance, and before long you'll get an 'I miss you' text begging you to come back. You need to decide right now what you will do with that text. If you reply, you will just reopen the can of worms and go right back to the start of the grieving process. Believe me, I've been there.

EXERCISE: GETTING CLOSURE

You need to get closure. Decide what your closure ritual will be.

- ♥ Write a letter to your ex but don't post it.
- ♥ Throw all his stuff in the bin. Even burn it if it helps you.
- ♥ Delete him from your social media networks, like Facebook or Twitter. What's the point in keeping him in your life?

♥ If you have mutual friends, keep each other at arm's length. You need time apart for your feelings to pass.

Moving on

How soon is too soon? How long is a piece of string? Everyone is different. If it was a bad break-up and you were dumped, you need time to heal, so just be good to yourself for a while. Spend time working on yourself and boosting your self-esteem, otherwise you'll just be vulnerable and make bad decisions. The trick is to stay mindful and measured going forward.

Relationships fail, but that doesn't mean that you're a failure. The only real failure in love is quitting. Or to put it another way, if you quit dating, you won't meet *anybody* – you're not even giving yourself a chance to fail. So keep dating. If you control what you bring to the table and keep going, an amazing man will walk into your life and will never want to leave.

The Dickhead Clearout

Okay, so dickhead is a strong word here. But let me tell you my own personal story and how the dickhead clearout has helped me to be happier.

I was going through a really tough time of it, as I had just buried a very good friend a few days before. When my ex texted, I thought he genuinely cared about how I was feeling and we arranged to meet up. I was still grieving for my friend and I thought my ex would be a shoulder for me to cry on. I should've known better when he said we should meet in a swanky bar in town – he was only meeting up with me for sex.

Seeing that I wasn't a barrel of laughs and that he obviously wasn't going to get any action from me, my ex started throwing eyes to another girl across the bar. By the time I was at the bathroom and back, he had made a connection with her and stayed with her for the rest of the evening, even kissing her in front of me. I walked out of the bar alone, feeling even worse than when I had walked in. He barely even said goodbye to me.

The next day he sent me a superficial text: 'Great to see you last night, you looked fantastic. See you soon.' I answered back and played along with his nonsense. 'Yes, great to see you too. Sorry for not being on top form.'

Over the next few days, I started to ponder the situation. I had actually apologised to him for grieving and for not being the sexy, bubbly girl that he'd wanted! After that, I started wondering why in the name of God I had decided to meet up with him in the first place. He didn't care about me or what I was going through, so why was I keeping him in my life? He had acted like a complete dickhead. He wasn't thinking of his grieving ex, friend or fellow human being. He was only thinking with his dick.

The story above is an example of someone in my life who was an energy drainer. Other examples could include a friend who suddenly drops you when she meets a man or the married man who's using you to escape from his life. None of them add anything to your life or invest in you in any way. They just make you feel bad about yourself in some way.

Once I realised this, I decided to fire some of my friends and so the dickhead clearout was born, aptly named after my ex. The dickhead clearout is an exercise to get negative people out of your life to make room for better, more supportive and positive influences. Simple.

The dickhead clearout gets you to be honest with yourself. It gets you to look at the friendships and relationships in your life to see if they are bad for you, then it gets you to do something about it to save you from years of misspent energy.

Life is a culmination of the things we do and the people we interact with every day. And if the people we interact with on a regular basis only have negative things to say, treat you in a negative way or make you feel bad or worthless or don't support your goals, then what chance do you have of achieving them? Look at your dating life to see if anyone is hindering your dating success. Are you investing your time in an unhelpful relationship that could be stopping you from meeting men?

Go back to the dating wheel on page 7 and ask yourself what your three most important focus areas are or the areas that you scored the lowest on. For example, if your self-esteem is low, ask yourself if there are people in your life who are contributing to your low self-esteem. Or perhaps the dating wheel shows that you haven't been on very many dates. Are you hanging out with friends who make it impossible to meet any new people? Do you need a new wingwoman?

Here are a few key questions to ask yourself to help you determine whether a relationship has become unhealthy.

EXERCISE: IS THIS A TOXIC RELATIONSHIP?

☐ Does your relationship with this person take more energy than it gives back?

☐ Do you feel bad when you're with this person or after you meet?

☐ Does this person laugh at your goals or offer no support when you ask them to?

☐ Does this relationship align more with their goals than yours?

☐ Do you constantly feel like you're not being heard?

☐ Do you have a mutually beneficial relationship or are you the one doing all of the giving?

☐ Is this relationship wasting your time?

☐ Do you have friends who repeatedly let you down at the last minute so that you end up staying in alone again?

☐ Is your ex still contacting you looking to hook up for a fling?

☐ Are married men in contact with you who are looking for a fling?

☐ Do you get sexy texts from random guys whom you briefly met looking for a fling?

♥ ♥ ♥

If you answered yes to any of these questions, you might have a toxic relationship on your hands or one that isn't aligned with your dating life. It's time to evaluate and deal with the situation or you will be stuck in a relationship that damages your self-worth and never have an opportunity to meet men.

Step one is to write down a list of five people who should go on the dickhead clearout. Give a reason why – the 'why' is the most important thing here.

EXERCISE:
YOU'RE FIRED!

1. Name of person: ....

   Why: ....

2. Name of person: ....

   Why: ....

3. Name of person: ....

   Why: ....

4. Name of person: ....

   Why: ....

5. Name of person: ....

   Why: ....

♥♥♥

Step two is to take action. Now that you have a list of unsupportive people in your life who are stopping you from meeting your dating goals, take action by applying the dickhead clearout methodology: either clear out, talk it out or space it out.

The dickhead clearout methodology

Clear out

Sometimes it really is necessary to cut off your relationship with someone entirely. You may have been picking up crumbs from a dead relationship for a while, an ex may continuously send you lame texts or a negative friend is a toxic presence in your life. It's time to let it go and move on.

In order to clear out, avoid any form of contact and stop communicating with this person if possible, especially with lingering exes. It may be helpful to remove them from various forms of social media so that you aren't tempted to reach out to them and fall back into old patterns. Remember your 'why'.

Talk it out

If you want to keep this person in your life or if they are someone who can't be removed entirely, one option is to try to talk it out. To keep things in line with dating, instead of constantly going to the local restaurant with the girls and sitting in the corner catching up on gossip, suggest trying the cool new bar where you've heard there are loads of men. Or if your friends are married, ask them to set you up on a blind date. If they aren't interested in supporting your plan, you will need to learn to space them out and not give them so much of your time.

Space it out

Family is forever, but that doesn't mean you need to let them hold you back from enjoying life and affirming your dating goals. Or if your dating life is at a low ebb, ask yourself if you have people in your life who support it. If not, what are you going to do about it?

Here's another example: many girls have a lot of gay friends. I know I do, anyway. But do you often find yourself dancing around a gay bar in the early hours with a better chance of meeting a Cher lookalike than meeting a straight single man? Of course I'm not saying you should ban all gay men from your friends list, but what I *am* saying is that you need to ask yourself if going to a gay bar aligns with your goal of meeting potential men. If not, you need to do something about it. It's like going to a sweet shop when you're looking for a steak. It doesn't make sense. Take a look at where you are spending your time. You don't have time to waste, so use it wisely.

Dating mentors

Oprah Winfrey said, 'Surround yourself with only people who are going to lift you higher.' Whether it's business, sports, relationships or just life in general, everyone needs a mentor. If you want to get better, you have to surround yourself with better people so that you can draw from their knowledge, passion and energy.

As you continue along your dating journey, you need to stay connected with people who inspire, nourish and bring out the best in you. You've got me already. I am right here with you, helping you and motivating you to be your best self and take control of your dating life. But you need more than me.

EXERCISE:
YOUR DATING MENTORS

Go back to the dating wheel on page 7 and ask yourself if the people in your life are aligned with your dating goals. Now think of at least one mentor for each part of your journey. For example, it could be a friend who's got your back, someone who gives you the motivation and the support you need but who also pulls you on up things that are getting in your way because they want the very best for you. Brainstorm your networks and write down as many mentors as possible for each category. If you can't think of someone, consider a professional in that field, such as a matchmaker, a dating coach, a stylist, a fitness coach, a nutritionist, a life coach or a therapist.

By spending time with these people, you will get the support and motivation you need to keep going. They may even be able to introduce you to a few good men along the way.

Dating wheel categories	Mentor(s)
Self-esteem	
Dating life	
Relationships priority	
Fun and creativity	
Social	
Packaging	

Move on

You don't have to change your friends, but you can change your focus and where you hang out. And don't let negative people rent space in your head. Make the decision to stay away from any people or environments that don't serve you and your goals. Only hang around people who help you grow and who are positive and encouraging.

All you need to do now is decide if your dating goal is worth it. Do you believe in your dream of improving your dating life enough? If you do, then the choice is pretty simple.

Over the last year, I have felt consistently happy. And during that time, I have cut a lot of people out of my life who dragged me down in one way or another: energy-zappers, promoters of bad habits, Judgemental Janes, rude people or just people who were on a different path than mine. Coincidence? Nope. Sometimes the best thing you can do for yourself and your bliss is to do a clearout so that you can move ahead.

Once you cut out or limit your time with people who are not supporting your dating goals, you will:

♥ Have more freedom
♥ Have more confidence
♥ Have better bonds with your truly supportive friends who will help you
♥ Attract more like-minded, positive people into your life
♥ Get better at quickly spotting negative people and cutting them loose
♥ Surround yourself with people who are in a similar place in life
♥ Have more time for yourself
♥ Learn new things and activities
♥ Have fewer arguments

- ❤ Do things that you really want to do
- ❤ Go places where you really want to go
- ❤ Be asked out more
- ❤ Have time to create more opportunities to meet men
- ❤ Have more wingwomen in your life
- ❤ Have more dates
- ❤ Feel better about yourself
- ❤ Have more fun
- ❤ Meet new people
- ❤ Be happier
- ❤ Reach your dating goals

I know a dickhead clearout sounds harsh, but it's one of the key steps in this book. If you keep choosing to put yourself in situations that are not aligning with your dating goals, you will lessen your chances of ever meeting anyone and you'll just be a people pleaser. You will be living someone else's life. Giving too much time to family, unsupportive friends, exes or deadbeat guys all takes a toll. Take off the comfort cape of your friends and family. It's time to take care of yourself and live your dating dreams. It's time to get centered and grounded and to reconnect with your relationship vision. You deserve the relationship you want.

Be brave. Be honest. You're ready for it!

Be the Flame

I used to think the old phrase 'like a moth to a flame' was fairly straightforward. Moths and flames. Simple. One remains in place, bright and beckoning, while the other flutters towards it with abandon, desperate to bask in its warmth and radiance.

'Be the flame, not the moth,' said Casanova. When you're the moth, you're always flying around from flame to flame and the world is filled with emotion. Moths are not in control. Instead, they hope, pray and dream about the flame.

And so the moth flutters all around the flame but never quite gets to it, and the flame always keeps the moth at a distance. But every now and then, the moth thinks there is a special connection with the flame and she dives in. Then the inevitable happens: the moth gets burned.

The moth backs away but now notices that other moths were circling around the flame that whole time, that others are being burned too and that more moths are showing up to replace them all the time. The moth flies away, with damaged wings and damaged pride.

Then one day, the moth spots another source of light and emotion overcomes her again. Despite the moth's better judgement, she finds herself inexorably drawn back, thinking *this* time it will be different. *This* time, the flame won't burn her.

The world of romance is full of moths and flames. Sometimes women are the moths, and sometimes it's men. But a skilled seductress will be irresistible to men. She will be the flame, and most of the men she meets will be moths.

Yet many women – even some of the most gorgeous women in the world – who haven't discovered their man-magnetising energy will continue to flutter around one flame after another, one date after another, and will keep getting burned. It doesn't matter how many dating books you've read, how many dating seminars you've been to or how hot that little black dress you bought is – if you are a moth, you simply don't get it and will continue to do the same thing over and over again until you burn out or just give up.

What do moths do in dating?

♥ A moth will keep sleeping with men in the hopes of having a relationship, and feel hurt and rejected when she's unable to get one.

♥ A moth will continue to chase any guy who shows her even the slightest amount of interest.

♥ A moth believes that against all the odds, she can rope a man into something long term, continuous and monogamous even if the man has explicitly said that he isn't interested in a relationship like that.

♥ A moth puts men up on a pedestal and fails to see their weaknesses.

♥ A moth is often addicted to the chase.

♥ A moth thinks a relationship will save her.

♥ A moth will still hang on in a friends–with–benefits relationship, hoping to convert it to something more serious, and will then judge herself harshly when it doesn't work out.

- ♥ A moth will enter into a relationship with a man even though she knows he's having dalliances with other women or even if he doesn't fit in with her value system.
- ♥ A moth will continually challenge herself to be the one moth that's able to bask in a dangerous flame's light without getting burned.

In essence, moths continuously hope for and chase after commitment. And when they don't get it and get shooed away, it's a real blow. Moths are mesmerised by men. They often think a certain man they have only just met has stepped straight out of the pages of a romance novel to bring them their happily ever after. These women are invariably disappointed when the night of passion doesn't lead to a *life* of passion. Moths have great expectations for every man they meet, far greater than the man wants to provide or even *can* provide. It's a vicious cycle.

Are you a dating moth? If you are, this cycle must stop right now. Decide here and now that you are the flame.

What do flames do in dating?

The flame has a certain glow about her, an aura of loving energy for everyone she comes in contact with. The flame takes charge of her own happiness and spreads her glow over every man she meets. But the flame also shields herself from anything that will weaken her. The flame protects herself from destructive dating patterns.

Look at your last five relationships or dating experiences. Were you the flame or the moth? And if you're thinking that you're neither, then I assure you that you were the moth!

Were you the moth?

☐ You do all the chasing.

☐ You tend to jump into things.

☐ You regularly fantasise about the relationship, even though you may have only just met him.

☐ You don't see the signs that he's not interested in you.

☐ He's always slow to text you back.

☐ You seem to be texting the guys more than they text you.

☐ You've had a series of first dates but never heard from the guys again.

☐ You continuously berate and question yourself when a guy isn't interested in you.

☐ You are in contact with a man who isn't suggesting to meet up at all.

☐ You are in a text relationship with a man.

☐ The man you like only texts you late at night.

☐ You have been seeing a guy for a while but just spotted that his online dating profile is still visible.

☐ You tend to suggest times to meet up with men rather then men suggesting times to you.

☐ You tend to suggest dating activities to men rather than men coming up with the dating activity.

☐ You often contact the man first after a date.

☐ Guys tend to treat you like an option and change their plans with you at the last minute.

☐ Guys always want to keep it casual with you.

☐ You've taken an ex back even though he cheated on you.

☐ You had a friends-with-benefits relationship but ended up getting hurt.

☐ You find yourself continuously thinking and fantasising about one guy.

☐ You will go on a date with anyone who asks you.

☐ You often feel vulnerable in a relationship.

Or were you the flame?

☐ You know what you want from your dating life.

☐ You concentrate on making your life amazing.

☐ You have many diverse passions and interests.

☐ You know that you are a great catch and deserve someone amazing in your life.

☐ You only invest in guys when they invest in you.

☐ You often have numerous men asking you out and you keep your options open.

☐ You never chase guys.

☐ You are generally so busy with your hobbies, your career and with dating other guys that you don't even give red flag guys the time of day.

☐ You celebrate men and enjoy men's company.

☐ You know that rejection is just part and parcel of dating.

☐ You treat yourself regularly.

☐ You celebrate the sexy, feminine, passionate side of yourself.

☐ You don't jump into things and you make mindful choices about your love life.

☐ You don't put yourself into situations that have the potential to hurt you.

☐ You don't blame men.

☐ You don't criticise men to your friends.

☐ You don't freeze men out (you are the flame, after all!). Instead, you are direct and open with men about your interests.

☐ You are often described as soft yet confident.

☐ You don't burn men and push them away with blaming words.

Now put a tick mark next to the statements above that ring true to you. If you ticked more moth statements, then you need to be aware that you have handed over control of your dating outcomes to someone else. You can't control someone else, but you can control you. Become aware of your destructive moth patterns and decide here and now to change. If you want to gain the power to meet amazing men, you must decide to be the flame. From now on, every time you feel hurt, crushed, disempowered or demotivated by a man, stop in your tracks and ask yourself: *Am I the moth or the flame?* By reeling yourself in, you will instantly start to make better decisions. And remember, when you decide to be the flame, remind yourself of its ability to protect you, give you strength and light up any room.

Eternal flame

A flame is soft and delicate, yet powerful, passionate, fiery and fierce, blazing with beauty. A flame is feminine, sexual, sensual, emotional, exciting, bold, brave and direct. A flame is confident and uncompromising and she knows what she wants. A flame has a feminine allure that draws men in and keeps them captivated for life.

A flame keeps burning regardless of a man's actions or behaviour and stays independent in her heart. She can deeply love a man and appreciate his affection and attention, but she won't put up with a man's crap and that's why she has no interest in taming bad boys. And the man knows that she will never give him too much emotional power, which is actually a major turn-on. When a flame uses the passion inside her as a motivation to be a better woman, going after her dreams and personal desires instead of directing it entirely towards a relationship, her man-magnet powers are perfected.

Get
Set

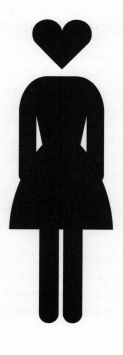

It's All About OTMs

You are reading this book because your networks are not working for you. You are not meeting potential men through your work, your social life or through the places you are going, so everything in this section is about three little letters: **OTM**, or opportunities to meet.

We've already established that you have to meet many men to find the diamonds in the rough. We've also acknowledged that if your social network isn't working for you and if you're wasting time doing things that don't align with your **OTM** strategy, then you need to do a clearout and surround yourself with positive forces in your life.

So where are all these great men? I get asked that question almost every day. Or I might get a question like this one: 'I'm a highly professional executive with no time and no desire to go bar hopping to find a quality man to have a relationship with, nor do I believe that bars are the place to go to meet a relationship-minded man in the first place. Where can I find the lifetime partner I'm looking for?'

The bad news is that there isn't one great place where all the single men congregate. But the good news is that they are everywhere. Men are all around you, but there is no way you are going to know if he's great or not if you don't go out and engage with them, meet them and date them.

In the following chapters, we're going to look at three networks and show you opportunities in each one of them. The three networks are the dating network, the personal contacts network and the out and about network. Let's get started.

♥

The Dating Network

Turn it on

Being online is now part of our lives. We shop online, pay our bills online, get our entertainment online and get our information online. Over the course of a few short years, social networking has gone from being the latest fad to being a core part of our daily routine. At a time when so much of our lives happens online, doesn't it just make sense that you have to incorporate the online community into your dating plan too?

Some people embrace the online dating world, but others will never give it a go. They say that they don't want their profile to be publicly displayed or that they've heard horror stories about it. One of the first things I ask a client who is hesitant about online dating is whether or not they are on Facebook. If they are (and not surprisingly, most are), I simply say 'welcome to online dating', since Facebook isn't that different to an online dating site. In fact, in the industry we see Facebook as competition. Facebook is nothing more than a social connection site (but now with loads of annoying ads thrown in) where friends and family stay in touch and easily exchange communication and photos. Or take LinkedIn, which markets itself as an easy way for professionals to connect – online dating sites market themselves as a social connection site for singles. Some sites target more elite clients, and their branding, price, the look and feel of their website and where they advertise (premium glossy magazines and business pages) all reflect a more affluent user. Other sites give a free service for a more one-size-fits-all approach. Plus new dating apps are being launched every day, so you can meet a new man with just a click or a swipe.

When people tell me they would never go online because there are only a load of loolahs there, it makes me laugh. Why on earth are they going on dates with loolahs? And what princes are they meeting in the alcohol-fuelled environment of the pub? The world of online dating is filled with the good, the bad and the downright ugly when it comes to suitors, so I'll just come out and say it: I can 100% guarantee that you will be contacted by undesirables. You will email them, swap numbers with them and you might even meet up with them. Let me tell you now that you will have to go through a lot of profiles, email a lot of men and even go on a lot of dud dates to potentially meet a guy you like. And even after all that, he might not like *you*! But that's okay; it's the nature of the beast. If that's the case, you don't want to waste your time with him anyway – you're looking for a guy who will prioritise you, remember? You need to accept that rejection is just part and parcel of the game.

But even though there are a lot of undesirables, it doesn't mean you can't control your fate. Much of your destiny online depends on the quality of your online dating profile, which means your written profile and your picture. Sub-standard profiles will attract any man. Great profiles will attract the best men.

Reel him in with your profile

This is your advertisement, not your daily journal! Men don't want to know your innermost feelings or your past dating woes. They also don't want to feel like they're being bought because your profile reads like a shopping list for a man's attributes.

Your profile is your opportunity to stop a great man in his online tracks and become the type of woman that he is willing to fight for – and by fight, I mean fight for your attention. This is your time to shine! It's time to write a positive, happy, flirty and fun profile that shows your strengths and interests but catches his attention and provides enough bait to reel him in.

But be aware that men struggle too. They might see your profile but can't think of something to say, get frustrated and consequently skip to the next one. Your job is to make it easy for him to message you. For example, if you just say you like to travel, well, who doesn't? It doesn't give the man any clear way to come back to you. During my days as a PR executive writing press releases for clients and submitting them to journalists, we always had to make sure there was a hook – a reason for the journalist to come back to us and eventually write up the story in the newspaper. So in the example above, let's say you change your statement to 'I'm an avid traveller and I have many interesting tales to share about my trips (don't forget to ask me about the time

I went shark diving!).' You see what you've done? You've just given him a reason to contact you by handing it to him on a silver platter and making it easy for him. All he has to do now is ask you about sharks.

Play with words to demonstrate how great you are. Use positive words such as *playful, smart, energetic, feminine, fun, flirty, upbeat, confident, fit* and *creative*. At the end of the day, quality men are attracted to positivity, not women who come across as disgruntled, too picky or desperate.

A picture is worth a thousand words

You have two choices: put up a picture or don't put up a picture.

Some people are hell bent on their privacy and don't want people to know about their personal lives, especially their relationship status. Perhaps you're afraid that you will see other people from work. Or maybe you have a job with a lot of authority or a job in the public realm. Politicians and TV presenters use my introduction agency service for that very reason, and confidentiality is key.

For everyone else, my view is: feck 'em! What's wrong with saying you're single? Don't forget, if someone saw you on an online dating site, it means they're single too! But if you still feel like you can't put your pictures publicly on the site, we can work with that. And even though you won't get as many clicks, you can control it more. You can hide pictures and offer them to men you're interested in after you exchange a few emails. But these pictures still have to be top notch and you still have to present yourself in the best possible way.

We live in an age where there's a camera in everyone's pocket, so people expect pictures. And if you're going to put up a picture, it needs to be damn good! I've been given out to loads of times about how superficial I am, but singles need to understand that visual chemistry is everything at the start, especially online. You're a fabulous person on the inside, but he doesn't know that because he doesn't know you – you're behind a computer screen, so all he has is your picture and your profile.

As a rule of thumb, you are only as good as your worst picture. That may seem harsh, but online dating can be a very shallow world. The standard of the pictures that people put up online is shocking. Remember, you're trying to lure a man, not use an online dating site for your latest holiday pics – put those on Facebook instead.

To get a better man, you need a better photo. Period. I have even sent some clients to a professional photographer, as no amateur can rival a professional for lighting and angles. Their job is to make you look good. There are loads of studios that also do your hair and make-up for a good price, and I highly recommend them. If you are low on funds it's a great present, so ask your friends to buy it for you for your next birthday. Believe me, it's worth it. Plus having your picture taken and getting your hair and make-up done for the shoot makes you feel wonderful and is great for your self-esteem.

Just one last bit of advice: corporate photos won't do! The guy has to imagine what you would look like on a date if he was to ask you out, so dress in date attire.

I recommend three pictures. A smiley, seductive head-shot is great as one of the three, but if you only show your face, many guys assume you're hiding something. The man wants to see the whole package. So how are you going to promote yourself? Look at your photos and ask yourself what that photo says about you. You may need to ask a friend for their opinion too. Be brutally honest!

Dos:

- Wear date attire.
- Feminine, sexy and figure-hugging dresses are best.
- Have at least three pictures. You can just use one photo and then offer the other pics to men you're interested in. Plus it will make them feel special that you are only sending this pic to them.
- Make sure your packaging is right – your hair, make-up, etc.
- This isn't surprising, but men really do prefer profiles of women who show cleavage. Your cleavage is part of your body, so you don't need to cover it up. Keep it classy, but a push-up bra can make all the difference.
- Understand your body shape to make the most of your assets and downplay your flaws. In other words, don't wear anything that accentuates your negatives – if you have bad arms, wear long sleeves.
- If you don't have a picture, get a professional photographer to take one for you.
- Stand out from the crowd with unusual jewellery or accessories, that picture of you with a celebrity or a photo with a cool backdrop.
- Most importantly, remember to smile!

No gos:

- Don't post a picture of you with a drink in your hand.
- Don't look serious, sad or corporate.
- Don't post a picture of you with a group of friends (they may in fact fancy one of your friends!).
- Don't post a picture of you doing sports. You aren't going to wear your tracksuit on the date!
- Don't post a picture of you with other men (men are turned off by this).
- Don't show too much skin – stay classy.
- Don't look bland.

Next steps

So you're online. You have the great picture and the eye-catching, buzzy profile. What do you do now?

I believe that men like to do the hunting in dating. It goes back to caveman times, and I'm not messing with the cavemen. But how is he supposed to hunt you down online if he doesn't know you exist? Other dating books say you should never, ever contact a man first online, that you must always wait for him to initiate contact. Well, I think that's bullshit. There is loads of choice online, which means there are loads of distractions for him and that there is a good chance that you will never pop up in his search tool. So what do you do? Certain dating experts would say leave it, that it's not meant to be or 'what's meant for you won't pass you'. But where does that get you? You'll just be left with all the undesirables that you don't even want to contact you in the first place.

Ladies, you need to man up a little. Grab the mouse with both hands and start clicking. Remember, you are doing the choosing, not waiting to be chosen. It's like joining a gym and looking at all the cardio machines but never actually getting on one. Hopping on the machine and using it will get you results, not just signing up for the membership.

A lot of sites have buttons to signal interest – use them! Sending winks, kisses, hugs, whatever are all web ways to flirt, and flirting is king. Initiate a conversation and get him to check out your stellar profile.

Here's an opening message for you: 'Hi X, you seem fun. I have a feeling that we will get on well. Perhaps too well… ;) Check out my profile and let me know if you would like to see more.' And so the emails begin.

Choice overload

Now that you're online, do you spend hours flicking through profiles? Do you have an extensive online check-list? Do you spend more time online than you do on actual dates? If you have answered 'yes' to any of these questions, then you may well be a choice addict.

When given so many choices, some people have trouble making any decision at all, and this indecisiveness could lead to a cascade of negative effects. In the book *The Paradox of Choice* by Dr Barry Schwartz, he writes, 'Choice overload can make you question the decisions you make before you even make them, it can set you up for unrealistically high expectations, and it can make you blame yourself for any and all failures. In the long run, this can lead to decision-making paralysis.'

Here are a few tips to overcome the choice paradox and harness the power of technology to your advantage.

Offline is better than online

There are two words in 'online dating'. The 'online' part is where you connect with someone digitally and the 'dating' part is where you actually go on the physical date. If you get stuck online, you are only doing one part of the process. Meeting someone in the flesh is way better than any computer interaction. I often find that people do the online part very well and send lots of emails back and forth ... but never actually go on any dates. But the date is the best part! Even if you don't have any chemistry, you can use the date as practice. The main thing is to keep meeting new people.

Tick tock – watch your clock

It's nice to open up your account and be inundated with messages and new matches, but you live a busy life. You have family, friends, work and hobbies – you don't have time to be stuck online in a fantasy life. The more time you spend choosing your partner, the less time you have to actually live in the real world. And ladies, I hate to bring this up, but you have a certain body clock to think of too. If you want to have children, you only have a limited amount of time to make that happen, so don't waste too much of it online.

Write a list

Although one day someone might invent the perfect algorithm to match two people, no online dating site has yet provided proof that its formula works, regardless of what its marketing department wants you to think. Don't expect the online service to find you your perfect match. There's no perfect mate out there, just people who you can enjoy spending a day – or maybe even the rest of your days – with.

You can streamline your options by making two lists. The first list should be the 'must-haves' and should include the attributes you require in a mate, such as age, education, looks, religious background or other variables. The second list is 'nice-to-haves' and consists of attributes you'd like in a partner but don't consider to be relationship deal-breakers. This approach will simplify the choice for you and cut out options that don't meet your initial needs.

Two site minimum

Internet dating can become addictive. I recommend using two sites at any one time. Just remember that being online is only one part of your dating plan, not your only search, so invest equal time in all areas.

Singles events

I'm not going to spend a lot of time on this, as singles events are self-explanatory and are, well, events for single people. Basically it's like a tradeshow where customers can go check out suppliers who are looking for business. At singles events, you know that everyone is single and you can meet people in a real-life environment.

There are numerous theme nights, from speed dating to lock and key parties to wine and food tasting mixers. The theme doesn't really matter – any theme is just a catalyst for communication or an icebreaker. Personally, I'm not a big fan of speed dating events. I find them to be too formal and they don't allow conversation to flow in a natural setting, but you might like this more structured approach. The trick is to be open and fun-loving enough to treat the event like a night out. This will give a man an idea of how you will act on a date outside of a themed event.

There are singles events going on every week all over the country. Research them and leave your inhibitions behind, and you can really enjoy your night out with other single people, irrespective of whether or not you fancy anyone there.

Professional matchmakers

Although online dating agencies and singles events are great ways to meet people, they fail to make sure there is a mindset match – in other words, what type of relationship the person is actually looking for. For instance, do they have time for a relationship? Have they dealt with past griev-ances? Do they have children, and if they do, how are they managing that situation? Are they looking for a long-term relationship or a casual fling? These are all questions that a matchmaker asks a potential client before they decide to take them on.

A matchmaker's job is to headhunt eligible singles who are genuinely looking for a relationship and make an introduction based on their criteria and interests. Matchmakers get to know you personally, co-ordinate dates and offer dating and relationship advice. A matchmaker basically manages your love life for you so that all you have to do is be available to meet your matches.

Even though this is the most expensive of the three dating options, a matchmaker can't make a man for you and there are no guarantees that you will meet the man of your dreams. However, it is definitely the safest and the most personalised method, as all members are screened and interviewed. And if privacy is key for you, then matchmaking is really your only option, as confidentiality is a selling factor.

Matchmaking isn't the be all and end all for everyone. For starters, it can't compete with the numbers from online dating, so there's always going to be less of a dating pool and thus less choice. Similarly, you can meet everyone at a singles event rather than just the one person a matchmaker introduces you to.

But how many hours have you wasted online messaging a guy over and back only to find out that he just wanted a one-night stand while you were looking for something more long term? Even at my own singles events where guys book online to come along, I never know what they are looking for. They may just be looking for a night out with fellow singles, or they could be starting a new job in a different country in a few weeks and are just looking for a casual short-term fling.

This is where the benefits of matchmaking can really play out. Plain and simple, matchmaking is for people who are genuinely looking for a relationship. By asking a series of questions in a personal consultation and getting clients to fill out a comprehensive application form, we are able to figure out their relationship mindset and hence introduce two people who are genuinely looking for the same thing. We take the hard work out of wondering is he or isn't he looking for a relationship.

It's all about connecting

Using dating services may sound intimidating, risky or even expensive, but let me put in a good word for the dating industry. Whether it's online, singles events or professional matchmaking, the goal is always the same: to connect you with a new person.

There are pros and cons to each facet of the dating world. Yes, there are bad eggs online, just like there are in the real world, but as long as you date safely and trust your gut, you will have more dating choices than ever. Yes, if you go to a singles event everybody will see you there, but who cares? After all, it just means they are single too. Yes, professional matchmaking is expensive, but if you're willing to spend money on that new handbag or the next holiday with the girls, then why wouldn't you also be willing to spend money on meeting a great man who you can share your life with?

Are all dating services for everyone? Probably not. Do they work as a whole? Yes, but not always. Whether you decide to manage your own dating life or let a matchmaker do the work for you, dating services may well find you a great guy.

♥

The
Personal
Network

What would you say if I told you that the people you already know – your friends, family and work colleagues – could be hiding the man of your dreams from you? You'd be pretty pissed off, wouldn't you? But that might be exactly what's happening! You have a better chance of meeting a great guy through someone you already know because he's been pre-qualified – he comes with a personal recommendation, and after all, your friend has your best interests at heart (well, at least we hope they do!). So let's start thinking outside the box and start brainstorming the possible opportunities for all your friends' friends.

Here are a few success stories from some of my clients.

Jenny, 28, wasn't meeting any potential partners at her work because everyone was too old or already married. However, through our brainstorming we realised that her friend Edel worked in a cool, young and dynamic web-based company. I set Jenny the challenge of making plans to catch up with Edel for drinks after work the next Friday to get to know Edel's work colleagues. She was honest with her friend about her intentions and Edel introduced Jenny to the single men who were out that night. Jenny met John, who was a similar age and had a similar zest for life. Jenny and John have been dating for three months.

Liz, 40, was an editor of a magazine. She regularly went out, but because of the industry she worked in she only met other women or gay men (sorry for the cliché here!). Through our work, we identified that her neighbour was a member of a sailing club and had mentioned that there were a lot of single middle-aged men in it. Liz didn't sail herself, but that didn't matter. I set Liz the challenge of joining her neighbour for Sunday drinks after the sailing had finished and to ask her neighbour to introduce her to any eligible men. She did it, and on the first evening she met Gareth, a friendly, divorced businessman. It took three Sundays for Gareth to ask her out, but they are currently dating.

All **Ruth**'s (38) best friends were married or in long-term relationships. Every second Saturday the girls would have a night out in town, which usually involved going to a fancy restaurant and drinking until the early hours, but the only men she would see were the waiters. I got Ruth to realise that even though her friends were married, they could still be wingwomen. So Ruth told her friends that she wanted to meet more men and asked if they knew anyone. At first they all said that they didn't know any guys who would be her type, but after she brainstormed with them a little and said she didn't care about types and was just interested in the opportunity to meet more men, her friend Carol suggested that they meet her husband and his friends in the local pub after dinner. Ruth met Matt and they hit it off straight away.

One way to take the pressure off your matchmaking friend is to ask them just to set up an opportunity to meet rather than a blind date. Blind dates can be tricky, even for the best daters. So get your friends to organise drinks, dinner parties or an activity where there are other people around and just invite you both along.

Also ask yourself if there is anyone in your life already who you have a bit of a thing for. I'm always surprised by how many people come to me when they already have a potential great man in their life but haven't done anything about it.

Gwen, 35, an attractive, smart solicitor, had decided to move her law practice from the city back to her hometown for financial reasons. However, the move would mean that she'd have fewer opportunities to meet men. Gwen stopped going out and concentrated on her business for the first year, shutting off any chance of meeting anyone in the country. She wanted to meet a great man and knew deep down that if she continued on this path, she would pack up and go back to the city before long, which really wasn't an option for her business. Besides, she actually preferred the country to fast-paced city life. We worked together for over an hour brainstorming ideas about how to re-energise her social life in her hometown and look for opportunities in her area. Gwen agreed to get involved in a local charity fundraiser to get to know more local women. Her brother was also involved in the local rugby club and had invited her up to the club for after-match events. She had always turned down his invitations, as she didn't want to be hanging out with her younger brother's friends. But the next time he asked, she decided to take the bull by the horns and she met her brother for a few drinks after games. It didn't take long for Gwen to meet Stuart, a handsome rugger bugger who had just been transferred from his job down the country. They took it slow and began to explore the local area together. They are still dating.

Rebecca, 32, complained that there were no single men left in town. Over the course of our session, it emerged that she lived with a great guy who she really fancied, but she didn't think it was appropriate to flirt with her flatmate. There she was, under the same roof as a guy she actually liked, but she wasn't doing anything about it! I set Rebecca the challenge of allowing herself to get into the flirt zone with her flatmate, Frank, and out of flatmate zone. Rebecca induced some chemistry by setting up a few romantic evenings in the house – candlelit dinners, some good music and a nice wine usually does the trick – and before long, they had got together. They dated for a while but realised they weren't right for each other. Rebecca eventually had to find a new flatmate, as it got too awkward with Frank, but at least she stopped procrastinating about her feelings and did something. You'll never know if you don't try.

Here are some more suggestions and questions to get you going:

- The next time your married friends have a dinner party, ask them to invite someone of the opposite sex along.
- Do you have a friend who is a social butterfly who seems to have better networks than you? Contact them and start to hang out with them. They make great wing people and they always know about the best parties in town.
- Throw a trash to treasure party, which is a fun way to clear out the stuff you don't want, pick up a few new treasures and meet some new people in the process.
- Organise a counter date – you set your friend up and they set you up.
- Go on a double date.
- Do you have friends who work in a more male-dominated job than you?
- Do you have friends who go to a lot of balls, social gatherings or other networking opportunities?
- Are any of your friends involved in sports? Can you go to any of their events?

EXERCISE:
TAKE ACTION

Brainstorm your personal contacts and write down at least 10 people who you think might know great men. If you are struggling with this, then write down the name of a friend, a family member or someone else who could help you with this exercise. The more people who can help you think outside the box and use your networks, the better!

Now write down the name of the person or activity, then write the action and steps you need to do beside it. I've included a couple of examples to help you get started.

Person or activity	Action
My friend works in a cool IT company.	I will ask to join her the next time she and her workmates go out for Friday night drinks.
My sister plays golf in the local club.	I will ask her if I can come along to one of the club's social events.
1.	
2.	
3.	
4.	
5.	
6.	
7.	
8.	
9.	
10.	

♥ ♥ ♥

♥

The Out and About Network

I'm always struck by the number of people who expect to meet someone by sitting at home. Who do they think is going to drop by? The pizza man?

If you don't naturally meet a lot of new people and you feel you have exploited the dating and friends networks for all they're worth, you'll still have to create at least a third of your new connections yourself. Remember, the reason you are reading this book is because your networks aren't working, and the only way to get your networks to work better for you is by going out there and interacting with other people. Simple!

The more places you go, the more people you meet and the more activities you take part in, the more chances you have of meeting not just men, but *great* men, since great men are usually those who live life to the fullest too.

Be your own entertainment officer

Over the next few months, make socialising a priority. Look at your diary and schedule at least two opportunities a week that you create for yourself. It's great to get invited to something and you should obviously say yes, but this is about more than that. I want you to become the 'inviter', the social hub, the entertainment officer.

Your challenge is to invite some friends or someone you know or a potential date to an event. But first, here's a tip: the word *date* can actually put men off. It takes a lot of guts to ask a guy you like out on a date. If I'm honest, I struggle with asking guys out on official dates too. But more than that, it can also make a guy flustered, as a date can come across as being too structured or arranged. And what happens if you've just met him and think he's cute but don't know him well enough to meet up with him on your own? Should you lose the opportunity to meet up with him so that you can test the waters to see if there is any chemistry? Of course not!

The challenge here is to create opportunities to *meet* men, not to create opportunities to *date* all men. So why not kill two birds with one stone and invite him along to a pre-arranged event with your other friends, which means that you'll get to catch up with your old friends while also creating an opportunity to flirt with this cute guy in a casual way without any pressure on either of you. So instead of asking the cutie on an official date, keep it casual at the beginning by saying, 'What are you doing Friday? There's a bunch of us trying out the new bar on the corner for happy hour drinks between 5 and 7pm. Come join us.'

If there is a connection, you can step up the flirting levels to more private flirting, and if there isn't, you can keep it to the more playful social flirting level, thereby avoiding any awkwardness whatsoever. He may even invite a few friends too, which opens up your networks even further.

So, invite, invite, invite. Every week, think of something that you can invite people along to. Make plans right now and start inviting people. The more, the merrier! Don't be afraid to invite a few potential guys to the same event. All you are doing right now is having fun and flirting. What's wrong with that? It's only when he starts investing in you that you start investing in him.

Olive, 38, married her childhood sweetheart, Tom, when she was just 20. If you believe in soul mates, then Olive and Tom were most definitely that. They were each other's first love and had never even dated anyone else. Olive had trained as a nurse and Tom was an engineer. His job required a lot of travel, so they had to move a lot to different areas if a project came up. Moving didn't faze them, as they were so enthralled with each other that they were happy anywhere and preferred to keep to themselves. They settled in one small town for a number of years, bought a house and lived a very happy and loving life together.

However, their happiness was cut short when Tom was tragically killed in a road traffic accident when he was only 34. Olive was devastated. The first year on her own was horrendous as she grieved her only love. Her family lived far away, and even though she loved them, she didn't want to move again and had invested in the home she had bought with Tom. She went from work to home, home to work, and she became lonely. Six months after his death, the friendly assistant in her local grocery shop, who had noticed her sad, heartbroken face, asked how she was doing and invited her along to a local fundraising dance. Olive declined and wondered why the assistant would say such a thing when she just wanted to be left alone to grieve.

A year passed and Olive's heart continued to ache, but she realised that she had no more tears left to cry. Coincidentally, around that same time Olive met the same shop assistant, Marie, who again invited her to a local festival. Olive found herself saying yes and agreed to go. It was the first time she had gone to an event without her husband. Olive felt insecure and outside her comfort zone when she walked into the local dance hall. But she needn't have worried, because Marie made sure she was introduced to her group and before long she was chatting to a few people on the night and even managed to laugh. The next day, Olive went down to the local shop to ask Marie when the next event would be on. Marie smiled at her enthusiasm but told her that there wouldn't be another town event for two months. Olive couldn't wait that long to engage with people. She had felt so alone for so long.

Olive invited Marie over to dinner as a thank you. It was the first time anyone had set foot in her house other than her family or Tom. Olive was a great cook and Tom had always told her that she should share her gift with more people. Olive cooked a feast for Marie, who was also an avid cook. The ladies giggled all night and shared their different recipes with each other. As she went to bed that night, she made a commitment that she would do this more often, with more people and with more food. And so Olive's supper club was born. Every second Friday, Olive hosted a dinner party in her house where everyone had to bring a new dish and a new guest. Sometimes there would be five people, sometimes there would be ten, but there was always loads of food and loads of banter.

Olive's supper club idea spread throughout the town and became quite the talking point. One time, her friend Karena brought Ken, the local vet, who was immediately taken with Olive's enterprising ways. Ken came back for another supper club, but this time on his own. Olive hadn't started the supper club to meet a man for romance, but she was flattered by Ken's advances and could feel a connection with him – something that she hadn't felt in a long time. Ken took it slow with Olive and eventually asked her to try a new restaurant in town with him. Olive liked Ken. She took a deep breath and opened herself up to a new love.

This is one of my favourite stories in the book. Olive learned to embrace her new life, even after tragic circumstances. Even though she was reluctant to at first, Olive took up her friend's offer (using her personal contacts network) of getting to know new friends. Then she went one step further and became the inviter herself to create opportunities for others to meet, and in so doing she met a great man herself.

Think about all the ways you could put yourself in a more social environment by exploring other interests, whether it's taking an acting class or joining a tag rugby team or taking a wine appreciation course. Remember, this is all about trying something new. If you've been going to the same pub every Saturday night, find a new pub in a different area or go to a new festival. *New* is the key word here, both in terms of trying something new and meeting new people.

Be a tourist in your own town

I did an interview with a journalist last year about why she gets approached by men so much more when she's abroad than when she's back in her own environment. She was shocked when I told her that it had nothing to do with the men and had everything to do with her and her mindset. When she was abroad, she was a tourist and was more open to new places to go and things to do. And because of that open, curious and friendly demeanour, more guys were attracted to her and found it easier to approach her. She wasn't rushing from appointment to appointment like she was back home; she was just taking in everything around her. Plus her cute Irish accent and her flaming red hair allowed her to stand out from the crowd, which helped too.

Think about how you act when you go on a city break. You want to learn as much as possible about the area, try the local restaurants and go to interesting places. But you don't have to go abroad to be a tourist – you just have to have the tourist mindset. Act like a tourist in your own town. There are always new restaurants and bars opening, and there are always new areas to explore and cool new things going on. That sense of adventure is one of the best attitudes you can have. Who knows what could happen?

So you've got yourself in the right frame of mind – now where do you go?

Pubs get a bum rap

Pubs and bars often get a bum rap as a bad place to meet a great guy. Having said that, though, it's true that they are full of players and guys who are looking for sex. But what guy *isn't* thinking about sex? Wouldn't there be a problem if he wasn't? And who said you have to have sex with him anyway? I'm asking you to create opportunities to meet men, not sleep with them!

In Ireland, a pub is much more than a place to drink and pick up a casual fling. The Irish pub lies at the very centre of the community. It's a place where people can drop in for drinks after work, where businesspeople make deals or entertain clients, where families gather to mark birthdays, deaths and christenings, and where sports fans go to cheer on their teams. Plenty of couples meet one another amidst the jolly chatter and clinking pint glasses of the pub. You don't have to go to a pub just to look for a hook-up or to drink yourself to oblivion. Mingle around, be friendly and enjoy the social nature of the pub scene.

However, when you are choosing a pub to go to, you need to start thinking like a man. I asked a recent client who was always out and who insisted there were definitely no men left in town to list the bars she was frequenting. Her list was full of the most upmarket wine bars, restaurants, cocktail bars and VIP nightclubs. Have a look around these places – there are usually more women than men, and if there *is* a man, he's probably there on a date. Of course, not all wine bars are like this; just try not to go to places that are too girly.

Sports bars or pubs are full to the brim with men hanging out with their buddies and watching their favourite teams playing on the big screens. Go to any sports pub near a stadium (soccer, GAA, rugby – it doesn't matter) on match day, and women will be outnumbered by at least 10 to one. Or go one better and buy a ticket to the game itself. Even if you're not interested in that particular sport, who cares? You never know who you'll be sitting next to, and you'll have the game to talk about later on. If money is an issue, just make sure you're in the pub for the pre- and post-celebrations and at least know the score and a little bit about the teams playing.

Just remember to have a balanced social plan. Pubs and bars are only one part of your third network, not the only segment. Scout out new activities and get ready for a new adventure. Create a lifestyle that brings people into your life.

Build your social plan

So let's get to work building your social plan. And remember, this is *your* plan. Do what *you* want to do, irrespective of what other people might think.

You'll see that I have also listed family events. Remember what we learned about using your networks? Your cousins, brothers or sisters may know a great man who's just right for you, so either ask them to bring him along or introduce you to other singles. Or just use this time to catch up with them and arrange a time to be introduced at a later date. Do keep the more manly stuff in mind, but it's always good to have a wingwoman on your side, so a few girly events aren't all bad.

Here are a few ideas to get the gears turning.

- ♥ Family events – do you have any weddings, etc. coming up?
- ♥ Dinners at your house
- ♥ Pubs/nightclubs
- ♥ Festivals (music, food, sports)
- ♥ Sports events (horse racing, rugby, football)
- ♥ Sports (gyms, running clubs, cycling)
- ♥ Classes (whatever you're passionate about – writing, acting, wine appreciation, dancing, cooking)
- ♥ Clubs (cards, poetry, public speaking)
- ♥ Meet-ups
- ♥ Seminars (personal development, holistic)
- ♥ New areas that you would like to visit
- ♥ Charities (fundraisers, balls, events, committees)
- ♥ Local events
- ♥ Networks
- ♥ Professional events (networking, corporate seminars)
- ♥ Current affairs (committees, fundraisers, seminars)

EXERCISE: BE A TOURIST
IN YOUR OWN TOWN

Brainstorm all the things to do and places to go in your area. Be as creative as possible here. Think about all the things you've always wanted to do but haven't got around to yet. Approach this exercise as if money and time weren't an issue. The point of this exercise is just to get as many things down as possible.

1. ....
2. ....
3. ....
4. ....
5. ....
6. ....
7. ....
8. ....
9. ....
10. ....
11. ....
12. ....
13. ....
14. ....
15. ....
16. ....
17. ....
18. ....
19. ....
20. ....

Now that you have a list of 20 things that you would like to do, take a look at the list you've made and pick your top 10. These are your top 10 action points for your social plan. But you can change this list from time to time as you learn more, hear about new things and make new friends. I'm always adding to my own personal top 10 list. When I started out, I hadn't a clue. I didn't know where to look or even what I wanted to do. But as my interests have become more refined, the activities that I want to do just pop up in front of me, so I keep adding them to the list. You might not have time to do all 10 right now, but the top five entries on your list are your five must dos that can't be procrastinated. This is so important that I want you to stop what you are doing right now, slot these into your calendar straight away and get out there.

EXERCISE: TOP 10

Activity	First steps	Date	Who will you go with?
1.			
2.			
3.			
4.			
5.			
6.			
7.			
8.			
9.			
10.			

If you remember nothing else, remember this

If you remember nothing else from this whole book except the three letters **O-T-M**, I will have done my job well. You must create opportunities to meet people – specifically, new single people, and even more specifically, new single men.

The man you want isn't waiting outside your door. He isn't going to stop you on your path and declare his undying love for you as you are rushing to work. I've said it before but I'll say it again: the reason you're not meeting men is because your networks aren't working for you. Your job is to get the wheels of your networks rolling again. The **OTM** strategy, if used correctly, gives you the framework to multiply your networks, either by using the dating services that are already out there, by using your friends' networks or by giving you the power to get out there yourself.

As you get out there more (both online and offline) – going to new places, meeting new people, accepting invitations to new events and becoming the ultimate inviter yourself – your dating life will reach new heights. You will feel more energised, you will be more interesting and people will react more positively to you. Everything begins with you. Only you can take control and create a winning **OTM** strategy. I promise you that if you do this, even just for a month, you will have opportunities everywhere and you will wonder how you can fit all the new men into your life.

♥

Playing
the Field

There are lots of good reasons to date several different men at once when you're beginning a new dating plan. If you feel alarmed by the thought of dating more than one man at once, the first question you should ask yourself is, 'Why?' You aren't committed to anyone. There is nothing wrong with exploring your options. Don't you think a door-to-door salesman would be pretty stupid if he invested all his energy on one potential sale in a new area rather than presenting his business to a few potential interested parties? You need to do the choosing, not wait around to be chosen.

Right now, it's all about getting out there and creating opportunities for yourself, wherever they present themselves. It's about meeting different people, spending time with them doing things you enjoy and potentially seeing them again. I want you to get outside your dating comfort zone and see the environment like I do, with an abundant single **MENtality**.

I'm not saying you should play the field forever, but at the start, right now, it's necessary. There are loads of single guys out there, I promise you that. However, there aren't loads of *great* guys out there or guys who are meeting your needs. But in order to find the great guys, you have to weed out the duds. It's like the door-to-door salesman – he has to knock on 10 doors to make that one sale.

The benefits of multiple dating are, well, multiple. We've all heard of feast or famine, right? The feast isn't just a coincidence – meeting and attracting amazing men happens to those who have an 'abundance' mindset. Plus keeping an open, multiple view on dating means you won't put all your eggs in one basket with one guy, which means you'll be less inclined to come across as needy or desperate with a guy that you actually like. Say you really hit it off with Paul on a first date and he wants to see you again on Friday night, but you're already booked on Friday night with a first date with Oliver and you're only free to see Paul on Sunday afternoon. Men love to see that a girl is busy – it presents a little challenge to them.

Get outside your comfort zone

I'm setting you a challenge that will get you outside your comfort zone: I want you to date the following five types of men at least once (feel free to add more). By creating more opportunities to meet different men who aren't your usual type, you will have a better chance of meeting the right guy.

1. The blind date

Love them or loathe them, blind dates combine mystery, suspense and surprise into a one-night-only experience and are a sure way to instantly get you out of your comfort zone. Pre-dating excitement is at an optimum and this can add to the chemistry of the evening. Ask one of your friends to set you up, or if you have the funds, go to a professional introduction agency. Fate is left up to the matchmaker, but it sure is a lot of fun.

2. The bad boy

Some say a bad boy isn't interested in true love, only quick love, but give him a chance. Bad boys tend to be assertive and will have more of an aggressive approach to the hunt for you. Since most women want a man to pursue them, this can be really appealing, as you don't have to wait too long for flirtations and initiations to develop. He may well treat you like crap and forget to call you again, but that's okay just this once because you are doing the choosing and you will keep going. Bad boys have been doing this for years – you'll just be playing him at his own game.

3. Your polar opposite

There's a reason why opposites attract – life would be boring if we were all the same! The chemistry between opposites is like magnets that are drawn together. Yes, you might have some avid arguments or differences, but if you step back from it a little you can learn a lot about yourself and maybe even bring something valuable to the other person's life too. Embrace this date. If you connect on values, morals and ethics but have polar opposite personality types, then you could actually complement each other and have a real chance of a relationship.

4. The younger man

Guys have been dating younger girls for years. It's time for women to start doing it too. Younger men often really like a confident older woman. You may even be able to show him a trick or two!

5. The silver fox

Every girl has dreamed about going on a date with George Clooney, or even better, Sean Connery. There's something worldly, experienced and shyly confident about the older man. More than that, older men often know how to treat you like a lady, not his plus one for his Xbox.

Invest in men like you'd invest in the stock market

Women are natural nurturers. We have an innate need to provide care and comfort to those around us. So it's only natural that you want to care for your man – invest your time in him, buy him gifts, help him with his problems, cook for him, sleep with him, contact him even though you haven't heard from him, reply to his lazy text message with an essay. But none of these things will make him fall in love with you.

In dating, the number one rule is **only invest in guys when they invest in you**. Too many women invest too much in one man without any investment from him whatsoever. Like our mothers used to say, 'Why should he buy the cow when the milk is free?' If he knows that he has you without question, your value goes down. Then he'll start to back off because he feels the desperation and bitterness that are brewing inside you because you aren't getting what you need fast enough and you start to become unattractive. And who could blame him?

Invest in men the way you'd invest in the stock market. Choose several men, like stocks, to invest a small amount of your emotions in. Then watch their performance. Until your investment proves its value, don't invest any more. Remember, *you* are a valuable commodity.

Multi-level dating

So many of us become 'lost' when we fall for a man and he becomes the centre of our world. And yet the moment we even *think* about a man as the 'centre of our world', his feelings of attraction for us go away. It may feel good to his ego, but it does nothing inside his heart. What makes a man go crazy for a woman is the fact that he might lose her. Doing your **SWOT** analysis (pages 52–53) will help you stay balanced so that you don't place him on an altar to worship.

But what if I told you that I had a system that eliminates all the uncertainty, struggle and hopelessness when you find yourself in a relationship that is going nowhere, dating men who suddenly withdraw or wondering why that one special guy isn't calling you back? What if the process of finding a fulfilling relationship could not only be effortless, but fun? What would it be like if you felt completely in control of your dating life?

Listen, I've been there. I know there's nothing more confidence-bashing than a man who doesn't contact you after a great date or who sends a lazy Sunday night text message or who doesn't seem to care how you're feeling. It can make you feel downright awful and unwanted.

But now imagine a dating life that always leaves you calm, cool and collected and where the man you are attracted to calls exactly when he says he will because he doesn't want to lose out on spending time with you.

Introducing the multi-level dating strategy!

Multi-level dating (**MLD**) simply means dating more than one man at the same time. When you are part of a multi-level dating strategy, you have full permission to flirt with as many men as possible without any fear of feeling guilty. Yes, that's right – I want you to flirt with as many men as possible. Online, face to face, anywhere and everywhere.

I started out my career in dating by running traffic light discos in college. Eager (and drunk) students would be stamped with a different colour depending on their relationship status. Back then, the colour green meant you were single and available. Red meant that you were in a relationship and unavailable, and orange meant 'maybe'. I never really knew what 'maybe' was – are you in a relationship or not? – but for some reason, everyone wanted to be orange. The purpose of a traffic light party is to decrease the apprehension associated with approaching potential mates at parties. It also provides an easy indicator of your unavailability to fend off unwelcome advances.

We're going to use the same traffic light system for multi-level dating, but in this case green is for guys you want to keep dating, orange is for those who you aren't sure about and red is for the men you are red carding for whatever reason.

Green = 3–8 dates. Only one man can be green. Keep dating if he shows promise, if you're attracted to each other, if he's genuinely interested in you and if you're starting to get exclusive. You'll probably have discussed taking your online profile down, introducing each other to family and friends and you might even be planning a weekend away together.

Orange = 0–5 dates. As many men as you like can be orange. You're still not sure and are not exclusive. He needs to prove himself more and invest in you more, but there's still the potential to be a great relationship.

Red = any number. The number is irrelevant. It could be one date or it could be 20 dates, but the point is that you have decided never to date him again.

If you are just starting out in dating, I want you to gather as many oranges as possible. You know that old saying, 'when life gives you lemons, make lemonade'? That's exactly what I want you to do, except this time, well, it's oranges. Keep dating, flirting and engaging with men and moving them up the multi-level dating system depending on their behaviour.

If you've had a few dates with a guy in the orange, he must either do something positive and move up to green, do something negative and get red carded … or do nothing and stay orange. There can only be one green at any given time, but also know that a green can be demoted to orange or may even be given a clear red. The clear red cards are the no gos – exes or people who do something that goes against your principles.

So what are the benefits of multi-level dating?

1. No more neediness

When you're multi-level dating, you have choices. You're not sitting around waiting for one man to call. You're having a blast meeting different people and doing different, interesting things every weekend. You actually start feeling more interesting and attractive because men see you this way.

2. It makes him want you more

It's a challenge to get you, which makes him want you more. He'll realise that there's a good chance you won't wait around for him to pull his act together and that he has to step up or risk losing you forever. Plus there are few things that are more attractive than a woman who has standards and knows what she will and won't put up with.

3. Drama queens need not apply

Men don't want any drama, especially at the beginning of a relationship. I want you to repeat this over and over again until it sinks in: no drama! Just one whisper of drama can take a great woman out of the game, so avoid it at all costs. But **MLD** takes care of the drama for you, since you're not banking all your feelings on one man. If you're afraid that if you flirt with or date other men then the man you are with will be upset, then you're missing the point of **MLD**. Making the *man* afraid is the whole point, but you want him to realise that on his own.

If you have just started dating a guy you like but he's not investing in you enough by not texting you back promptly or arranging more dates, you don't need to tell him what's he's doing wrong – **MLD** will do that for you, as you'll be so busy with the guys who *are* investing in you. In fact, it will turn *him* into the drama queen, as he'll be fighting for your time, your attention and your love.

4. The world is your oyster

By using your **OTM** and **MLD** strategies, the world is your oyster and your stage to be the most attractive, desirable and sought-after woman you ever thought possible. The more you date, the better you become at it.

MLD in action

Multi-level dating has been a transformational dating tool for my clients. Are you wondering how it works in practice? Let me give you an example.

Sorcha had had three dates with Will. They had a lot in common, but he had already cancelled two dates and he was being a bit lazy about the whole thing. Even though she liked him, she was starting to think that he needed to up his game.

Sorcha had bought tickets for a cool burlesque show and asked Will if he wanted to come along. He said he'd love to, but a few hours before the show, he showed his true colours when he called to say that he had forgotten to organise a babysitter for his son, whom he has every second weekend (from a previous relationship). Red flags started to go up. How can you forget to organise a babysitter? Will said there was nothing he could do, but he wanted to make it up to Sorcha the next day. She just said, 'That's a pity, but cool, let's have a coffee in the next few days.'

Sorcha hung up the phone, disappointed that her Saturday night was now ruined. She sat on the couch, mulling it over. Should she stay in and watch a romantic film in desperation or should she ring a friend and offer her the ticket? But she had wanted her Saturday night to be a date. But here's the thing: because Sorcha was using the **MLD** strategy, she was able to go on Tinder and send a message to Scott, a guy she'd communicated with a little. She said, 'Look, I know this is a bit random, but my date for tonight just cancelled and I have tickets for a cool burlesque show in town. I could ask a friend to go, but I think you're kinda hot, so I thought why not? Are you free in an hour?'

To cut a long story short, Scott said yes but he did point out that he didn't like the fact that he was her second choice. They had a great first date. They chatted all night and really enjoyed themselves. Sorcha's Tinder date was now the frontrunner, and boy was he hot. They had so much to say and so much in common. They went on another two dates and both of those times were fantastic too. On the fifth date, Scott told Sorcha that he liked her, but he wasn't looking for a relationship right now. The thing is, though, Sorcha really liked him.

So there she was on a fifth date with a man who wasn't sure. She could have tried to convince him what an amazing person she was and how happy she could make him, but because she was still using the **MLD** strategy, she simply said to herself, 'He can take all the time he wants to come to a decision about us, but he can't have me all to himself while he's mulling it over!'

So instead, Sorcha focused on making herself happy. Knowing that she had the **MLD** strategy to fall back on ensured that she was as cool as a cucumber about the whole thing. She bumped Scott back to the orange level and carried on. He would only be put in the green area once he proved himself and showed that he wanted to invest in her. Sorcha filled up her calendar with other activities and she still went on dates with Scott, but he didn't get the same attention from her, as she was genuinely busy.

Two weeks later, when they were on their eighth date, Scott told Sorcha that he really liked her and that he wanted to be exclusive with her. Three months later, they're still dating and it's still as good as that first date.

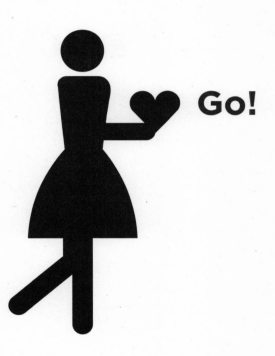 Go!

♥

You Are
a Goddess

Dating can be overwhelming sometimes. We need to multi-task our careers and our dating lives more than ever, master the online dating technology and deal with the visual world that we live in, not to mention trying to pick the great guys out from all the less desirable ones. Sometimes we can lose our focus and direction and get sucked back into our destructive dating patterns.

So where do you find the strength to keep going? Where do you find the inspiration to be so irresistible that guys will fall at your feet? Where do you find the insight to make the right decisions? No one technique or book will help you here if you don't have the basics right. When you close this book, you'll be out there in the dating world on your own and you will need to make your dating decisions yourself.

Why techniques don't work

My dating coaching style is different than most. I did a TV interview on *The Saturday Night Show* with another well-known male dating coach from a pick-up artist school. He constantly talked about techniques and how learning off a series of routines and chat-up lines can 'pull' any girl. That's not how I operate. I don't think there is a one-size-fits-all technique. Getting better at a routine will give you more confidence, but what happens if that particular routine doesn't work? What do you do then?

I have always empowered my clients to work on their state of mind first, and that philosophy hasn't changed. All techniques flow from your state of mind. If you get that right, the rest will fall into place.

When asked how he prepares his team for a big game, the manager of my hurling team, the mighty Tipperary, was quoted in a newspaper as saying, 'It's a question of whether you put structure before instinct or instinct before structure. Hurling is such a quick game and it is difficult to theorise about it. I like instinct. Players are encouraged to move, encouraged to solve their own puzzles. Some days it works, some days it doesn't... There's only so much you can do for players. You have to allow them to play a little bit and make sure they have the confidence to do it. We do try to encourage where they should be and where they shouldn't be, but it has to come from within.'

The same goes for dating. There are only so many techniques or routines you can learn, but if you don't have the right state of mind or good self-esteem, it will all be for nothing. We've been working on getting you out there to meet more men and to give up your bad dating patterns, but it has to come from within. Your instinct will help you to make the right decisions rather than letting techniques guide you up the garden path, which only leads to a dead end.

But I believe in you, and I believe you will find a great guy to have an amazing, loving relationship with – and I believe that your instinct will guide you. The secret isn't flicking through this book – or any book – trying to find the killer move. The only way to achieve your goals is to go back to basics and build a foundation of beliefs and values that are so strong that it will give you the power to flirt, make great dating decisions that are good for your soul and allow your true beauty to dazzle any man. This foundation is what I call your goddess self.

Rocking your goddess self in dating is all about embracing essential elements like self-esteem, beauty, femininity, sex and independence. Getting in touch with these elements will give you all the tools you need to access your inner goddess and let her shine.

There is a strong debate as to whether irresistible women are born or made. It can actually be both. Some women have an innate sensual goddess presence, but most of us have to learn as we go along, and those who do learn to embrace their goddess powers have men falling for them, chasing them and treating them well.

Goddesses throughout history

What is it about Angelina Jolie that brings men to their knees? Why is Helen Mirren the thinking man's fantasy? And what on earth can we learn from Camilla Parker Bowles about keeping a man in sexual thrall?

Throughout history, there are tales of irresistible women who have effortlessly lured men and cast them under their spell. There are women who walk into a crowd and instantly stand out, women who are as alluring as they are dangerous, women who captivate men with tempting desire. And the truth is, every woman wants to be like them.

Cleopatra is one of the most fascinating goddesses who ever lived. Two thousand years after her death, there are nearly 200 films, TV movies and documentaries about her and almost 4,000 books. The story of Cleopatra and Caesar began when Caesar set his sights on her native Egypt. In order to save her country, she had herself secretly delivered to Caesar in a rolled-up rug to seduce him with her beauty and charm. Let's just say that when Cleopatra tumbled out of the unfurled carpet in front of the 52-year-old general, she made a big impression and Caesar fell madly in love with the courageous Egyptian queen.

Other examples of goddesses are France's most famous diva, Édith Piaf, Coco Chanel, Madonna, Demi Moore, Elizabeth Taylor and the Duchess of Windsor, who had a man give up the throne of England for her. And then, of course, there's Marilyn Monroe, my favourite goddess.

Modelling Marilyn

What is the exact cocktail of irresistible traits that makes Marilyn Monroe the ultimate goddess? And what lessons can we learn from her that we can apply to our own lives?

Be the ultimate flirt

If there was an actual science to flirting, Marilyn would hold the highest degree in this field of study. She flirted with her co-stars, she flirted during press conferences and most of all, she flirted with the camera. She could flirt with the entire audience and yet still somehow make each person feel like they were the only one she was flirting with. Marilyn used everything she had to flirt – she flirted with her eyes, her hips, her tone, her lips. She also had a real gift of using flirty banter to create playful intimacy. In one press conference, when asked what she wore to bed, Marilyn replied, 'What do I wear in bed? Why, Chanel No. 5, of course.'

Let yourself shine

Many people who worked with Marilyn or knew her personally spoke of her luminescent energy and the light that she radiated. But we all possess this inner light. Think of a time or night out when you were positively radiating. Step back into that memory and remember how you felt and how people reacted to you. This energy is who we truly are on the inside, suddenly made visible to others. Marilyn knew how to turn on her light so bright that men would think she was the only woman in the room. This glow is simply irresistible to anyone in the near vicinity, but when you shine that light onto another person, it's more powerful than any other trick or technique there is.

Embrace your sexual side

Marilyn almost single-handedly started the sexual revolution of the 1960s, which was no mean feat. She put a new twist on sexuality. It wasn't dirty, shameful, shocking or embarrassing – it was fun. She made no apologies for the fact that sex is enjoyable, and not just for men! In an interview, Marilyn said, 'I am invariably late for appointments, sometimes as much as two hours. I've tried to change my ways but the things that make me late are too strong, and too pleasing.' Men love a woman who embraces her sexual side. It's not about being a slut, it's about unleashing your inner sexual goddess and delighting in your entire sexual being.

Stand out from the crowd

Marilyn was the original when it came to turning a scandal into an opportunity. Paris Hilton and Kim Kardashian look like they ripped the pages right out of her book, but unfortunately skipped past the sections on class and charm.

In 1952, in a sexually repressed America, Marilyn's career took a nosedive when a nude calendar of her started appearing in gas stations across the country. The photos were from a shoot she had posed for years previously and they were now making her a household name. Marilyn responded to the scandal head on with her special brand of humour. When asked what she was wearing, she joked, 'It's not true that I had nothing on … I had the radio on.' And when asked why she posed nude, her honest answer was one everyone could understand: 'It paid $50 and I needed the money to pay my rent.'

I'm not telling you to create a scandal or pose naked just to stand out from the crowd. What I *am* asking you is to step out of your comfort zone and take some risks, and even better, sexy risks. Sure, you might make mistakes and you might end up with egg on your face, but turn it around and make it fun.

Be vulnerable

I can't think of anyone who was more vulnerable than Marilyn Monroe, which has made her fan base as much female as male. She tried to live her life with no regrets and she saw beauty in her imperfections and mistakes. She said, 'I believe that everything happens for a reason. People change so that you can learn to let go, things go wrong so that you appreciate them when they're right, you believe lies so you eventually learn to trust no one but yourself, and sometimes good things fall apart so better things can fall together.'

Vulnerability is about feeling *all* your emotions. Letting your vulnerabilities come out allows you to be more in tune with your emotions and more connected to other people and to society in general. By removing the blockages and really feeling and being honest with your vulnerabilities, you can experience the courage to truly love. We all have many reasons to protect our hearts – heaven knows Marilyn had plenty of reasons too. But take chances, embrace your vulnerabilities, feel the fear and do it anyway.

Embrace your femininity

Marilyn was all woman! She used her femininity in her sexy, sultry voice, she used her womanly curves in her style and even the wiggle in her walk screamed femininity. Marilyn enjoyed her femininity, and you should nourish and celebrate your feminine side too. Embrace your femininity and really be the woman that you are. In doing so, you will stand out and make men want you more. Feminine qualities are things like sexiness, softness, patience, sweetness, empathy and affection. Choose a few feminine qualities and experiment with them. Take a practice makes perfect approach and watch your love life change for the better.

'You don't have to be beautiful to turn me on'

The biggest misconception about goddesses is that they are all incredibly good-looking. You don't have to be drop dead gorgeous to be irresistible. Like Prince said in his song 'Kiss', 'you don't have to be beautiful to turn me on'. At first glance this seems like a simple line, but coming from Prince, who was known at the time for dating the most beautiful women in the world, it's a shocker. Yes, looks and all the visuals are the first things that catch a man's eye, but the deeper qualities are what make him stick around.

Maybe you have a friend or know a woman who by any standards is quite plain to look at, yet her whole being has a kind of goddess quality that projects the conviction that she is a raving beauty. Alluring yet mysterious, confident yet feminine, she is always in the company of men. She also has individual traits that heighten her appeal. Perhaps she is exceptionally smart and creative and wows men with her mental agility. She is always beautifully dressed and expresses her sexual self, yet she remains elusive. Maybe you've watched in awe as many a man has been driven to wild acts over her.

Through such women's example, I began to understand that while it helps to be beautiful, it's not essential to being irresistible to men. And besides, beauty alone is never enough. Men are most attracted to women who are convinced of their own goddess qualities and appeal. These women live large, as if men and life were created for their pleasure.

These goddess qualities are the foundation that we need to build on. Each woman can create her own signature brand with her own series of individual quirks, tricks and talents that personalise and heighten her appeal. But first, we need to identify the qualities that make goddesses so alluring and then make that foundation rock solid. The following chapters look at some of these goddess qualities, which are a blueprint for bringing out your own.

A goddess knows that a relationship doesn't equal happiness

Goddesses embrace life and go with the flow of love, but a goddess knows that a relationship doesn't define her. A goddess doesn't need a relationship to make her happy.

The gravitational force of a goddess will always lie in her appeal, her power and the energy that she exudes and radiates. It is her effortless charms and her confidence that make the world take notice of her. As you work on developing your own goddess, stand back and watch as the world takes notice of *you*.

♥

Sexuality Is a State of Mind

A sex goddess embraces and owns her sexuality. Being a sexually expressive woman is about being balanced, sensual and intimate. It's about being *alive*. Sexuality isn't about having big boobs or the perfect pout. Sexuality is a state of mind.

A sex goddess has achieved a state of mind that radiates a strong aura of sexuality without having to do much. Actually, your mind is also a sexual organ, but in order to truly maximise it, you need to become confident as a sexually expressive woman. Basically, you have to understand what sex is to you before you can express it. Your sexuality is a physical, organic and functional part of you and it's hugely important in our discussion about dating.

Every relationship, no matter how fairytale romantic it may be, has a core of sexual attraction. Even if you prefer to take things slow and build up trust and emotional intimacy before escalating to a physical level, you have to acknowledge that any relationship that is going to move beyond platonic friendship is going to have a sexual element.

A lot of my clients forget how important sex is in a relationship. When I probe them on the subject, they say that they don't think that they deserve pleasure or they think it's not that important. They talk about relationships like it's just something to do – they want a man to go to the cinema with them, go to family events with them and sit in on a Friday night with them. But more often than not, they forget to mention that they deserve a man to have great sex with.

Ladies, sex is a big deal in a relationship. It's not the only thing, of course, but it's a big thing, and anyone who doesn't think that way needs to stop kidding themselves. You deserve to be with the most amazing man, have the most amazing relationship and indulge in the most amazing sex – and you have to be open to all three.

I've been coaching women for a long time now, and the thing that seems hardest for women to do is to find ways to *authentically* feel more sexual. Many women want to know how to look more sexual to men, but many have never felt real pleasure or know what it is. They say, 'Look, I just don't think I'm that sexual' or 'I don't know what turns men on.' If you want to be a true sex goddess, you need to be a woman who enjoys pleasure, and the first step is to open your mind to the idea that it's possible.

Ask any guy what one of the sexiest things a man can see is, and he'll tell you that it's a woman enjoying real pleasure. Showing a man that you are a great lover before you even start to date him will drive him wild. So stop worrying about what that one article in that women's magazine said about how to give great oral sex or stop worrying that you don't think you have enough experience with men. When you start doing whatever *you* want and get really excited in the process, you will please a man no end. Simply knowing this will help you ooze sex appeal.

An active imagination can do wonders for your dating life. Start thinking up loads of sexy thoughts with him in them. For example, when you meet a man, be open to the idea that you could have multiple orgasms with him. That might sound crazy, but being open to fulfilling your sexual desires in your mind is the first step to making those orgasms a reality.

Now, it takes some work to get to a place where you feel sexual and able to unleash your sexual side, both in and out of the bedroom. Like I said, it's really hard for women to authentically get to this place. And before we talk about some ways to make this happen for you, I'll re-emphasise the *authentically* part. You see, this is something that you can't fake. A woman must unleash her sexy side from within. A sexual goddess knows that the key to attracting a man is her sexual energy. It's the part of her that loves sex and knows exactly what turns her on. Because when a woman knows that, there is something just so damn sexy about her. A woman who knows what she likes in the bedroom and is open to new pleasures has a certain aura about her that drives men wild without her even having to say a word.

Top 10 tips to increase your sexual energy

I know so many women who don't know what pleasure is or who can't tell me a single time when they were turned on. How can you be sexy if you don't know what turns you on? For women, an orgasm is mainly a mental thing, but as long as you have a vagina and a brain, you have everything you need to experience an unbelievable amount of pleasure. But if you think you have a low libido, you have to do something about it — not for your potential man's sake, but for yours.

1. Treat your sexy self

Let's start small. Do something that makes you feel good about yourself. For me, a manicure and pedicure makes me feel pretty and feminine. When I first get my hair done I always feel fab, but my ultimate favourite is spraying on some Chanel perfume. It instantly makes me feel sexy, feminine and sensual.

EXERCISE:
TREAT YOURSELF

Write down 10 things that make you feel special and sexy. It doesn't have to be expensive, but whatever it is, make this exercise all about treating yourself.

1. ....

2. ....

3. ....

4. ....

5. ....

6. ....

7. ....

8. ....

9. ....

10. ....

2. Dress sexy

I love to use clothes and accessories to feel sexy. There are certain styles of clothing and textures of fabric that make you feel fabulous when you walk down the street in them or when you walk into a bar. I love leather fabric and I love my knee-high boots. They make me feel wild. I also have a sexy LBD that I team up with red lipstick that just screams sex goddess. And don't forget a naughty piece of lingerie. Nobody knows you're wearing it, only you, and that's all that matters. My favourite piece is my suspenders. Wearing them always gives me a naughty little glint in my eye because I know something that no man does!

Go through your wardrobe and pick out 10 pieces of clothing that make you feel sexy. If you don't have any, flick through some magazines for inspiration or ask a friend for a loan of a dress that you saw her in that you thought was hot. Whatever it is, you need to have a few key items that you can wear that will instantly transform you into a sex goddess.

3. Get a sexy photo

We can all flick through magazines and admire the sexy celebrities, but it can also make us critical of our own bodies. But the good news is that with the right make-up and professional lighting and posing, we can look every bit as beautiful as the models and celebrities in magazines. All you need is a great photographer and a few touch-ups to reveal your sexy self.

I'm a big fan of boudoir photography because they are tasteful, sensual photographs that capture a woman's femininity, sexiness and beauty. A professional boudoir photographer usually provides professional make-up, hair-styling and sexy outfits and will even show you how to pose. The results are always amazing and guarantee that you will look like a sex kitten by the end. And the best part is that you get to keep these photographs afterwards, so when you're getting ready for a date that you're feeling a little nervous about, you can take this photograph out and remind yourself of your sexy potential. Use the photographs like a switch to get back into the way you were feeling that day to instantly feel sexy, confident and feminine again.

4. Your bedroom is your sensual shrine

I'm a bit messy, but I make sure my bedroom is pristine. Make sure bed lockers are dust free and light some candles so that there's always a nice scent in the room. And nothing beats clean, crisp sheets when you jump into bed. A sex goddess needs a relaxing place where she can fantasise.

5. Love your sexy body

How can you allow your body to reach levels of ecstasy when you don't love your own body, connect with it, or worse still, berate it all the time?

Exercise will not only give you more energy and make you feel better about your body, but good cardiovascular health means that blood will flow better to all the pertinent areas. Massage is another great way to connect with your body, as it increases body awareness and reduces tension. You can do DIY versions, which you can personalise to make you feel more sensual and desirable.

Here's a sensual body appreciation exercise that I use regularly.

EXERCISE:
LOVE YOUR BODY

What you'll need

- ♥ Sensual, meditative, classical or jazz music
- ♥ Candles
- ♥ A hot bath
- ♥ Sensual scents – vanilla, ylang-ylang, lavender
- ♥ Body oil

Set the mood for some sensual alone time. Light some candles and play some relaxing music. Take a long, hot bubble bath with aromatherapy oils and soak for about 20 minutes. This will help to quiet your critical mind. This isn't the time to exfoliate or shave. Just relax.

Then, when you feel relaxed, get out of the bath and massage your body with your oil. (I love coconut oil myself.) Caress each part of your body and feel the textures and temperatures of different areas of your skin. Enjoy doing this for about 10 minutes, giving equal attention to each part of you while repeating the following words aloud or in your head: 'I love my body and I honour all its beauty.'

The first time you do this exercise, you might feel a little awkward. If you find yourself getting distracted by your thoughts, just go back to an area of your body. Some women find this exercise to be quite emotional, as it might bring up some past feelings or perhaps you have never been touched like this or said these things about your body. If you need to cry, cry. Just don't beat yourself up for not loving your body in the past.

Do this exercise as often as you can – at least once a week at the start. We are all so busy rushing around that we don't appreciate how much our body does for us and how beautiful it is. We should love it, not reject it for not being perfect. A sex goddess loves her body and all its imperfections.

6. Fantasise

Contrary to what the nuns may have taught you, thinking about sex isn't going to get you in trouble. In fact, it can be just the thing to help get you in the mood. Spend five minutes each day imagining yourself in your dream sexual situation with a gorgeous man. When you're on a date or just with a man you like, stop thinking about your to do list or wondering if your hair is okay and stop fretting about what happened in work or what he thinks of you. Allow your mind to wander to your pleasurable fantasy place and imagine having ground-breaking sex with him instead.

EXERCISE: FANTASYLAND

Write down a sexual fantasy that you have or would like to have. Perhaps it's having mind-blowing sex with a celebrity or even a friend in a unusual place. Be as descriptive as possible, using all five senses: sight, touch, taste, audio and smell. Remember, nobody will see this, only you, so allow yourself to get into the moment.

....

....

....

....

....

....

This is your go-to sexual fantasy. You might not be able to find the celebrity, but otherwise what are you waiting for?

7. Change the tune

A few years ago, my boyfriend broke up with me and I was devastated. I spent days locked in my room listening to Adele on repeat in floods of tears until something snapped and I could cry no more. So I decided to change the tune – literally.

Music has a profound effect on our mind and hence our behaviour. Music can enrich your life in so many ways and get you in the mood, but it can also do the opposite. It can bring back bad memories and make you depressed too.

What music turns you on when you're heading out on the town? What songs instantly make you feel sexy, fun and confident? You know, the song that makes you want to dance whenever you hear it, even though you were feeling wrecked before it came on. For example, the songs that instantly make me like a sexy, confident woman are:

- ❤ 'It's Raining Men' – The Weather Girls
- ❤ 'Girls Just Want to Have Fun' – Cyndi Lauper
- ❤ 'Brass in Pocket' – The Pretenders
- ❤ 'All the Single Ladies' – Beyoncé
- ❤ 'Born This Way' – Lady Gaga

Next, think about the same exercise but for times when you're relaxing and feeling sexy at home. For example, my favourite relaxing, sensual songs are:

- ❤ 'Let's Get It On' – Marvin Gaye
- ❤ 'La Femme d'Argent' – Air
- ❤ 'Come Away with Me' – Norah Jones
- ❤ 'Je T'Aime … Moi Non Plus' – Jane Birkin and Serge Gainsbourg

EXERCISE: CHANGE YOUR TUNE

What songs get you in the mood for a night out?

1. ....

2. ....

3. ....

4. ....

5. ....

What songs make you feel sexy when you're staying in?

1. ....

2. ....

3. ....

4. ....

5. ....

❤ ❤ ❤

Make a playlist of these songs so that you can instantly allow yourself to be serenaded by the tunes.

8. Study time

You can never stop learning how to be better at something. If you wanted to be better at cooking, you'd buy a cook-book or sign up for a class. If you wanted to be better at golf, you might take some private lessons. So why is there such a taboo about learning how to be better at something that connects so many parts of us? There are many tasteful, women-friendly books on how to have great sex out there. You never know what you'll learn and it will turn you on just by reading it.

9. Self-pleasure

The Big M – masturbation. There, I said it!

Look, I'm morto talking about this too. I'm blushing here, as I'm imagining my parents reading this. But we need to talk about self-pleasure and its role in looking for love.

There are many reasons why a woman could be celibate for extended periods of time. Age will have a part to play here, as the hook-up culture isn't as prevalent for those over 40. Or a woman may have come out of a loveless, sexless marriage that lasted way too long. Or maybe she's so scared of being rejected for her cellulite thighs that she keeps finding excuses to keep her clothes on and misses out on potential good relationships just to avoid getting naked. I have clients who come to me looking for love who have been celibate for over 20 years. Some clients who come to me have never had an orgasm.

But the longer you go without stimulation and feeling sexual, the harder it will be to go for it when it does come along in the form of a loving partner. So what can you do about it?

Well, I've been reading up on self-pleasure lately. There are so many positives about pleasuring yourself, especially if you don't have a partner, that it's just plain silly not to. Consider this:

- Self-pleasure can improve your mood.
- Self-pleasure and self-love can unleash your sex goddess within all by yourself.
- Self-pleasure can relieve tension and stress.
- Self-pleasure has proven health benefits.
- Self-pleasure can help if you can't sleep.
- Self-pleasure will help you learn what turns you on.
- Self-pleasure will help you to be more in tune with your fantasies.
- Self-pleasure will give you an amazing orgasm all by yourself.
- Self-pleasure will give you control and freedom.
- Self-pleasure will help you be a step ahead when you find a partner.
- Self-pleasure will make you a better lover.

♥ Self-pleasure will make you more likely to climax during intercourse with a partner.
♥ Self-pleasure will make you feel wonderful.

See what I mean? Not only can self-pleasure help you get in the mood, it can also improve your mood!

Remember when you were younger and a new toy always cheered you up? Apply the same theory to your sex life and get yourself a new (or your first!) sex toy. Don't laugh! The excitement of a new item in the bedroom will instantly make you feel saucy. Sex toys aren't hush–hush anymore, and there's something for everyone. Using a vibrator, for example, is a common way for women to learn how to achieve orgasm.

Pleasuring yourself keeps you glowing with powerful female energy and it makes your sexual self come alive. To be a confident, sexy woman, self–pleasure is a valuable and necessary part of a healthy sexuality that just so happens to be fun and feels good too. So go ahead and get to know yourself a little better. You'll be glad you did.

10. Talk to a doctor

Finally, if you're still struggling to feel sexually confident, you might want to talk to your doctor. There are lots of things that can affect your sex drive, such as birth control pills or antidepressants, menopause or a testosterone level that's too low (yes, women have testosterone too – surprise!).

Whether it's reading romance novels or erotic short stories, learning more about tantric teachings or even allowing yourself to experience the Big O more often, there are countless ways of getting in the mood and expressing your sexual goddess self. Whatever it is, find a way of making yourself feel like a sexy, sultry woman more often so that you'll always be smoking hot, even when it's cold.

♥

The
Flirtation
Formula

Goddesses are experts at the art of seduction. They know how to bat an eyelash and get that twinkle going in their eye, but they also know the serious side of physical intimacy and how powerful it can be when bringing a man closer. They love to flirt and banter and make eyes with men, giving them 'come hither … but only if you dare!' glances under heavy lids. Goddesses never stop flirting.

Flirting can be one of the more pleasant and exciting parts of life. It can make your heart beat faster and it can be the start of an unforgettable adventure. And I'm sorry to have to say it, ladies, but when a guy first approaches you, he's not thinking you look intelligent or like you have a great sense of humour – he's approaching you because he wants to see your clothes on his bedroom floor. Guys initially think with their 'little heads' and they'll fall for the simplest flirtatious sexual innuendo.

The good news is that you hold all the power in this initial meeting. His fantasies come from the mannerisms, gestures and subtle cues you send him, and yes, these are sexual. So for every flirt you send his way, the more he'll be motivated to approach you. My objective here is to give you the flirtation formula so that you can then unleash your intelligence and inner beauty that will make him fall in love with you.

The power of the flirt is not in its mannerisms, but in the fantasy it creates in a man's mind. The key to successful flirting is all about creating desire.

But first, in order to be a good flirt, you have to stop being so *nice*. Too many women are trying to do this whole butter-wouldn't-melt-in-their-mouth routine that is getting them nowhere while the sultry flirts are having all the fun. Veer towards being a little more risqué and you'll get a lot better results.

It's all in the eyes

Actress Tara Reid said, 'I can make a scene that's not supposed to be sexy, very sexy. It's a power you're born with. It's not a physical thing, it comes from inside. It's all in the eyes.'

Flirting begins and ends with eye contact. Eye contact is incredibly powerful, so it's important to walk the line between subtlety and intensity. Even from across a crowded room, you can signal your interest in someone merely by making eye contact and attempting to hold your target's gaze for more than one second (not too much more, though, or you'll seem threatening). If your target maintains eye contact with you for more than one second, chances are that he might return your interest. If after this initial contact your target looks away briefly (everyone does) and then looks back to meet your gaze a second time, you can safely assume that he's interested.

If you've been making eyes at each other for a while but he still hasn't come over to you, here's a trick that I learned from another dating coach that works great in bar scenarios. The next time you see a man you're attracted to, instead of doing the usual thing and wait for him to approach, or maybe doing the coy little smile or looking down at the ground and doing nothing, I want you to unlock your sex goddess.

I want you to look him in the eyes and imagine that you can give him the best damn blow job he's ever had in his life. Imagine that you can take this man and bring him down to his knees instantly. Look at him as you're picturing that and let your eyes say it all. What will happen now is that you will begin to smile and maybe even blush, but your eyes will remain primal – and he's going to look at you and he's going to feel that. He's going to wonder what you're thinking, and he'll be dying to find out. And oftentimes he's going to immediately feel attracted to you because there's intrigue. And all of this without you ever saying a word. If he's gutsy, he might even walk over now and ask you what's making you smile. You obviously aren't going to tell him what you're thinking, but you can simply say, 'Oh, I just thought of something hot', and it will make him go wild.

Smile like you mean it

My friends always ask me why so many guys come over and approach me. I'm no supermodel, but the answer is simple: I smile. I can't count the number of times I've been at a bar staring at a hot man across the room, and just by sending over a simple smile, he knows the interest is mutual. This then gives him an incentive to come over and introduce himself.

Both men and women often feel intimidated or worry that they'll get shot down, so they don't risk introducing themselves. But by smiling, you can take away this fear and make the sexy stranger even more interested and at ease.

Here are just a few good reasons to smile:

- ♥ Smiling makes you approachable.
- ♥ Smiling makes you adorable.
- ♥ Smiling is contagious.
- ♥ Smiling makes you feel good.
- ♥ Smiling relaxes you.
- ♥ Smiling keeps you positive.
- ♥ Smiling is a natural drug.
- ♥ Smiling makes you confident.

The best advice I ever heard about smiling was to smile at others the way you want them to smile at you. Remember, nobody wants to go on a date with Miss Misery Guts. And really, how can you look sexy, happy and irresistible if your face is tense? But it's more than that. You need to mean it. Men can spot an insincere smile a mile away, so connect with your inner sex goddess and let her help you smile from the inside out.

Teasing talk

If your mind is full of pleasurable, sexy thoughts, then your tongue will be too. Playful, teasing talk is a great way to make men attracted to you and to generally have a lot of fun. But there are ways of doing it well and ways of doing it badly. I've done both, so I'll try to save you some of the social pain I've endured trying to get it right.

One of my clients who had been on three dates with a guy but still hadn't even got so much as a peck on the cheek was afraid it was veering into friends zone territory. She emailed me to ask me what to do. I told her to send him this message: 'Just hopped out of the shower and thinking of seeing you later on. It will be fun!'

Let's break this down. You haven't said anything rude, slutty or out of line. All you've said is that you just got out of the shower and are thinking of him. But do you know what you've done? Knowing that men are visual, you have just created the vision of you getting out of the shower, and his mind is now racing, imagining what you would look like naked. You are also presupposing that the date will be fun, so before you've even seen each other, you have already created a fun, sexy experience. Bingo!

Start to use words that have hidden innuendos. Use suggestive language that implies sex without being explicit about it. It's a game that will keep your guy guessing. There are so many words that have a suggestive tone to them – words like *hot*, *sexy*, *naughty*, *cheeky*, *adventure*, *bold*, *steamy*, *fire*, *trouble*, *passion* or *bad*. For example, rather than saying, 'You look so nice' (who wants to be nice anyway?), say, 'You look really hot tonight.'

Try some of these on for size:

- ♥ To the work colleague you have a crush on: 'It's a good thing we work together, or you and I could get into a lot of trouble.'
- ♥ To the stranger with a beard: 'I love a man with a beard. There's something so primal about him.'
- ♥ To someone who's checking you out at a bar: 'I can see devilment in your eyes. You may need to stay away from me. This could be wild!'
- ♥ To a guy you're talking to online about your hobbies: 'I have a real sense of adventure. It can get me in trouble sometimes!'

❤ To a guy on a first date: 'You're bad! Quit looking at me
like that. You're giving me ideas and they're totally inappropriate right now.'

Or you can use your environment to describe what's
around you in a teasing away. It's that simple. For example,
when talking about your drink to the hot barman, rather
than saying it's a refreshing fruity cocktail, say, 'This cocktail
is so good, it's making me tingle all over.'

Put sexually surged words into your interactions with
men and you will see immediate results. Once you start to
use teasing talk in your conversation, he will start to tease
back, so remember not to go over the top. The essence of
flirting is the push–pull: you give a little, but then you pull
back. The magic lies in your imagination and your willing-
ness to be bold, daring and good-humoured.

Be as Pretty as Possible for Destiny

What's on the outside does count. Men are visual and fall in love with their eyes first, so looking your best is a must. A goddess knows that if what's on the outside looks just as great as what's on the inside, your glowing personality will surface effortlessly to let men see how fabulous you are.

Unfortunately, a lot of women don't get this and think that looks aren't that important. They think their inner goddess is enough to make a man come running over. As time marches on in the relationship, those qualities will almost certainly keep him interested. But we're focusing on the initial attraction here, and a lady's obvious physical strengths, not the ones hidden beneath her shiny exterior, will dominate the initial attraction.

Research shows that within the first 15 seconds of meeting a man, a woman will have subconsciously decided whether or not she will give him a chance to try to make her fall in love with him. In the same amount of time, a man will have decided if he is turned on by how a woman looks. Despite our lofty notions of appreciating someone for their personality, not their looks, nature has programmed us to select and respond to stimuli as sexually compelling or repelling simply based on good reproductive sense so that we can pick out who is best suited to carry on our genes and legacy.

While women use visual, emotional and safety (including financial) cues to assess a man's desirability, over 90% of a man's decision at this stage is purely based on visual cues. You have to maximise your appearance and you have to enjoy looking the best you can at all times. As Coco Chanel said, 'I don't understand how a woman can leave the house without fixing herself up a little, if only out of politeness. And then, you never know, maybe that's the day she has a date with destiny. And it's best to be as pretty as possible for destiny.'

Look good, feel good

Now before you go off saying I'm really superficial (and I have been called that before), as a professional matchmaker, I listen to what men want on a daily basis, and I am telling you that looks are a deal breaker when a man first meets a woman. I can't tell you how many male clients say to me, 'She would be just right if she lost a few pounds/dressed up a bit/didn't look so haggard.' Focusing on and enhancing the best aspects of your image will do more than boost your chances in the love market – it will also boost the way you feel about yourself.

The more effort you put into your looks, the better you will feel and the more he's going to compliment you – which will make you feel even better. It becomes a wonderful upward spiral. Look good, feel good. Feel good, look good.

Think of it this way too: when you meet a guy on a date and he has made an effort with his appearance and is looking good, there is an unspoken agreement that you have both invested some time and energy into this, which is one of the first stepping stones in a relationship.

On the flip side, don't get hung up on your physical flaws. Don't compare yourself to other women all the time and certainly don't obsess over the models' bodies that you see in magazines. How can you unleash your sexy self if you are constantly fretting about how you look? How can you celebrate your femininity and your beauty if you are always trying to look perfect? Perfectionism is not the same thing as striving to be your best. Perfectionism is a protection shield, since trying to be perfect or just like everyone else often leads to inaction: 'If I had the perfect nose, like Mary down the road, all the boys would be after me.' Like, really? As Rick Warren says in his book *The Purpose Driven Life*, 'Those who follow the crowd usually get lost in it.'

Here are some simple tips and tricks to look your best.

Liven up your looks

Everyone wears black these days. Sure, it's chic and it can hide a multitude of sins, but it can also be boring and un-original. Add bright, bold colours to your wardrobe or use accessories to add a talking point.

Here are five easy ways to liven up your looks:

1. Use colour in your wardrobe.
2. Wear interesting jewellery. Quirky earrings or an unusual necklace can be a great ice-breaker.
3. An unusual coloured handbag can liven up an outfit.
4. Try a different hairstyle. If you usually wear your hair up, leave it down and people will start commenting on it.
5. Brightly coloured lipstick will draw attention to your lips.

Dress for dating success

Virginia Woolf said that clothes 'change our view of the world and the world's view of us'.

Your clothes are one way you can show the world your goddess self. Go through your wardrobe and look at each item. Do your clothes make you feel sexy, confident and comfortable? I'm even talking about your gym clothes, your PJs and your underwear. Send any clothes that don't make you feel this way to the charity shop. What's the point of keeping clothes that don't make you feel good?

If your wardrobe is now bare, you'll need to hit the shops. Look for clothes that make you feel like the sexy goddess you are. Men are drawn to women who are comfortable in their own skin – and their clothes – and know how to show it. Everyone has desirable features that they want to accentuate and features they would like to tone down. Take a good hard look at yourself in the mirror or ask a friend what your three best assets are, as this will help you make good wardrobe decisions. For example, one of my best assets is my small waist, so I wear dresses and tops that accentuate my waist, which in turn draws attention away from my larger hip area. Marilyn Monroe did something similar with her famous white halter neck dress, which put the focus on her great cleavage rather than her size 14 hips.

If you're a novice to fashion or feel that style isn't your strong point, bring a friend along with you to go shopping, but be clear that you aren't necessarily going to follow the trends – you're shopping for clothes that will bring out the best version of yourself. What looks good on one person might not look good on another body type.

There are four main female body shapes: apple (round), pear (triangle or bottom heavy), hourglass (curvy) and rectangle (also known as straight). The styles of clothing that look great on an hourglass figure won't necessarily flatter a pear-shaped or an apple-shaped woman. Figure out what shape you are and then try to find clothes that will flatter it.

Many department stores have fantastic free fitting room services or personal shoppers, or better yet, enrol in a styling course to learn some basic styling tips from an expert. Resist impulse buys or a 'this will do the job' attitude. Take your time and don't buy for the sake of buying. Ask yourself if the item helps you to look and feel like a goddess.

And don't forget the lingerie! Knowing that you have a sexy pair of lingerie underneath your clothes instantly makes you feel more sensual and powerful. But lingerie can also give an extra oomph to your assets. If you've got it, flaunt it. And if you don't have it, then fake it with some great fashion fixers. For example, padded push-up bras can magically add a cup size or more and will enhance your cleavage with tops with a lower neckline, and shapewear will create a flattering silhouette under a figure-hugging dress. There are loads of options out there and the staff in the lingerie department are used to helping women just like you, so make the most of what you've got.

Beauty is skin deep

Cleopatra was renowned for her radiant skin. She bathed in milk to keep her skin soft and beautiful, and legend has it that she needed 700 lactating donkeys to supply the milk for her daily bathing regime. I'm not saying you should go out and milk donkeys, but you do need to have a good routine for your skin, especially your face.

Your skin is one of the most sensitive parts of your body, and regularly touching the skin all over your body is incredibly sensual (try the exercise on page 183). A man who simply brushes against a woman's soft skin can instantly get turned on.

Here's a natural skincare tip: using coconut oil is a wonderful way to make your skin soft, radiant and healthy without buying pricey cosmetics. Include a spoonful of coconut oil in your diet, use it as a moisturiser or indulge in coconut oil for your massages.

As for make-up, a goddess has mastered the art of the 'no make-up' look. Remember that the primary purpose of make-up is to perfect and enhance. In fact, many men are turned off by too much make-up. The goddess look is all about showing off your glowing skin, accentuating your luscious lips and allowing your sexy eyes to smoulder. Balance is key in make-up, so if you're concentrating on creating a sexy lip, keep the rest of your face naturally radiant with a bit of blush, a slick of shimmery, neutral eye shadow and mascara, and that's it. Don't overdo it – leave the theatrical make-up for those who are actually on stage.

Watch your waist

I know you've heard it a thousand times before, but exercise and good nutrition really are the best ways to feel and look great. You know the drill. If you sit on the couch every night watching TV, you will continue to fuel the habit of comfort eating. But when you exercise, your body wants to eat healthily, and when you eat healthily, your body wants to exercise.

Feed your body with nourishing food that will help you glow, food that's fresh, healthy, unprocessed, low carb and high protein. Find an exercise routine that feels right and make it part of your daily routine, be it yoga, Pilates, cycling, trips to the gym or long walks in the park. Just think of how much better you feel after a hike rather than sitting indoors surfing the internet or watching TV. If you think that men won't notice those extra pounds you put on over

Christmas or that you've hidden your bulges under that big woolly jumper, think again.

You might think it would be boobs or ass, but men get more excited about your hip to waist ratio than anything else about your body. Women have always known this, hence the popularity of the corset. Focusing on a flat stomach through core exercises (sit-ups, ab crunches) or at the very least through shapewear or a simple cinched belt around your waist will show off your feminine curves.

Keep your beautiful self shining

When a man locks eyes with you for the first time, he's locking on to your visual presentation and you want him to see the hot, beautiful woman that you are. And remember, if you are on date five or more, don't think you can get a bit slack in the visual department. He was turned on initially for a certain reason and he hasn't suddenly forgotten that, so be sure to keep your beautiful self shining.

♥

Confidence
Is Key

'When a woman becomes her own best friend, life is easier.'
Diane von Furstenberg

I'm afraid of so many things. I'm afraid every time I do a TV interview. I'm afraid when I have to talk in public. I'm still afraid of driving around the city. But if I carry around these fears and insecurities wherever I go and allow these fears to own me, how would I live my life then? I'd always be scared, paralysed and insecure. I'm only mentioning myself so much here because even though I show my positive, feminine, fiery side to you in the hope that it will help you, I struggle too. Everyone does!

So what can I do? Should I give up? I will never give up. Why? Because I have confidence. And the truth is that if you don't have confidence, it doesn't matter what techniques you learn, what man you start dating or what fabulous new dress you have. Confidence is everything. If you have confidence in yourself, you can do anything.

Here are three foolproof ways to make sure you are always a confident goddess.

1. Manage your state

In neuro-linguistic programming (NLP), a state basically means your mental state, such as whether you are relaxed, focused, motivated, bored, confident or any combination of such states. Controlling these states is the basis of NLP state management. Out of everything that I have learned from NLP, I have found state management to be the most powerful because most of my clients' issues are state dependent. Put simply, my clients were allowing an unhelpful and unproductive state to control them rather than choosing a more resourceful or useful state to get better results. To give you some dating world examples, I've had clients clam up in a state of nervousness on a first date even though they had been chatty and open with me in the consultation; clients who were in a 'reserved' state on a night out and then wondered why men never approached them; and clients who were in an 'unsexy' state and couldn't understand why men didn't find them attractive.

In all of those examples, the client had told me about times in their life when they felt confident, chatty and sexy. But when they went on the date, they had chosen to go into an unhelpful state that not only wasn't going to get them any results, but was going to make them feel bad about themselves, which would then cause a more negative state than what they had started off with. Can you see the problem here?

I want you to repeat after me: **I am the creator of my own thoughts.**

Once you realise that you create your own state of mind, you will see that you can choose what feeling to have on any given day. This doesn't mean you are devoid of emotions. It means that you are in control and that you have options. Know that you are empowered to choose your emotion or state and that how you choose to engage with, respond or react to something is all up to you.

I'll always remember my first big-time interview for a top TV show. It was called *The Saturday Night Show* and was on a prime Saturday night slot, hosted by Brendan O'Connor. My parents were in the front row and I could feel that they were anxious for me. I thought I was completely fine about the whole thing, but as I walked from the green room to backstage, I started to think of the lights, the cameras and one of the most controversial TV hosts in the country. My heart started thumping and my hands started to get sweaty. The TV researcher could see the look on my face and asked if I was okay, but that just made it worse. I was in a full-blown state of nervousness.

I knew there and then that being nervous was going to be no use to me going on a live TV show with a live studio audience. It wasn't the most 'useful' way that I could come across to the audience, come across on TV and engage with the host if I wanted to be memorable in the right way. I needed to take control and find a more useful character to be in. So in the few moments before I went on stage, I quickly thought of three ways that I would like to come across as. I thought that above all I would like to be seen as someone confident (who went out there and just did the interview), fun (who laughed and told funny stories) and flirty (who harmlessly flirted with the host, because how could a dating expert not flirt?). Then I quickly thought of an actress who embodies those three adjectives, and for some reason Reese Witherspoon came into my head. Using her as an anchor to focus my thoughts, I channelled the actress and stepped into her character in order to be fun, playful and confident, walked on stage and smiled at Brendan with a little glint in my eye as I told my story.

Or to give you another example, I've often been in a bar with my boyfriend after a long day in the office and have started to become distracted by my to do list or by thinking about the different clients I'd seen that day. But when I catch myself doing this, I ask myself, 'Is being distracted or in a state of worry about clients or your financials the most useful state that you can be in right now?' Then I quickly think about my main anchor, Marilyn Monroe, and I step into character, allowing the sexy, confident and playful parts of my personality to come out instead. My boyfriend won't know what I've just done, but he'll have a much better time in my company now.

Channelling your favourite actress or sex symbol can instantly change your mindset and help you to get into your desired state for a given time. You don't have to keep it turned on the whole time. Even sex symbols have some down time, watching a rom-com in their PJs with a cup of tea. The difference is that they know how to turn it on at the right time, and you can too.

EXERCISE:
PLAY THE PART

Who is your favourite actress? List three adjectives that describe her. Is she soulful, sexy, strong, funny, adorable, kooky? Whatever she is, write down a time you were each of those three adjectives.

1. ....

2. ....

3. ....

Now ask yourself how this actress would handle your dating life. What would she do? How would she act? How would she dress? What would she smell like? How would she handle men in general or a particular man that you like?

Write it down.

Repeat this exercise any time you're not in the most useful state you could be in. The more you do this, the more you'll start to feel like a sex symbol yourself. Trust me, this really works!

In dating, there are a series of states that work time and time again. But don't just take my word for it. Think about a friend of yours (or another celebrity if you can't think of a friend that fits the bill) who is successful with men, a bit of a goddess. Maybe she's married now, maybe she's still dating or maybe she's in a relationship with an amazing guy, but she always has men interested in her. Now look at the states listed below and put a tick next to the ones that she demonstrates when she's in the company of men.

Open	Feminine	Seductive
Fun	Flirty	Stylish
Sexy	Friendly	Inquisitive
Confident	Cheeky	Good listener
Engaging	Risky	

Now what if I told you that 80% of the people reading this book picked pretty much the same states? It means that there are patterns in what the successful daters do to get results. If you choose the more successful states instead of letting the unhelpful states override you, you'll get results too.

As a matchmaker, I can tell you that all men are looking for a woman with as many of the above states as possible. When I set up an introduction, I need to make sure that the woman will step up and encompass the desired states. After all, I can bring a horse to water but I can't make him drink. In other words, I can present you with a great opportunity, but if you're not bringing your A game to the date and instead choose unhelpful states like extreme nervousness, closed-mindedness, self-consciousness or wearing boardroom clothing, well, you might as well stay at home. Remember, you control your state; the state does not control you. You do the choosing. Learning to consistently put yourself in your best state is one of the greatest gifts you can give yourself – and your date.

2. Find proof

I know that you are capable of meeting a great guy. I know that you are capable of making a man fall at your feet. I know that you are capable of mesmerising a man and being so irresistible and sexy that he wants to be around you all the time. The thing is, you need to believe it too.

Go through each of the states listed below and any other ones that you think are useful in dating and write down at least three examples of times when you demonstrated it. For example, for the 'open' state, you might say something like:

♥ I was open to new adventures when I travelled through India.
♥ I was open to a new love when I met my current boyfriend on Tinder.
♥ I felt open when I talked to my best friend who I hadn't seen in ages.

Open

Fun

Sexy

Go Get Him!

Confident

....
....
....

Engaging

....
....
....

Feminine

....
....
....

Flirty

....
....
....

Friendly

....
....
....

Cheeky

....
....
....

Risky

....

....

Seductive

....

....

Stylish

....

....

Inquisitive

....

....

Good listener

....

....

If you don't have many examples of one particular state, think of something that you could do this week where you could demonstrate the state. For example, if you're struggling to find past examples of being sexy, you could run a hot bubble bath for yourself or buy some sexy lingerie. Or look at your **SWOT** analysis again on pages 52–53 and focus on all your strengths. The more proof you have that you've achieved these states, the more confident you'll become.

The next time you practise any of these techniques and a man looks at you – and I assure you that he will – I want you to instantly realise it and acknowledge it by saying something to yourself like, 'Wow, did you see how that guy just looked at me?' If you can show proof to your inner critic that you are in fact capable, your critic will shut up. Keep complimenting yourself and stop missing the opportunities.

3. Be your own best friend

You can practise managing your state until the cows come home and you can find every last shred of proof out there that backs up how amazing you are, but if you don't have the final piece of the confidence puzzle, none of it will matter.

This last piece is what most confidence coaches miss out on, but it pretty much sums up this whole book: you need to love yourself.

I'm a 100% self-loving devotee of myself. I'm my best friend and my biggest fan. I even fancy myself and think I'm really hot sometimes. Now before you think I'm barking mad, know that goddesses love themselves the most too. I can't stress this enough. Once you have this down, everything else will flow from it, as all your decisions will come from this foundation.

On a scale of one to 10, how much do you love yourself? Your answer to this question will dictate everything else. Look at it this way. The person you will be with the most in your life is yourself. When you wake up in the morning, you are with yourself. When you're lying in bed at night, you are with yourself. When you're walking down the street, you are with yourself. Even when you're on a date, you are still with yourself! What kind of person do you want to wake up with first thing in the morning, walk down the street with and see at the end of the day before you fall asleep? Because that person is you, and it's your responsibility to be the person you want to be with.

You need to make good choices for yourself that will make you feel good, not just immediately, but for the long term. I don't know about you, but I want to spend my life with someone who knows how to let things go, who feels safe, who's fun to be with, who laughs and smiles, who's sexy and carefree – and who loves herself, warts and all. So I need to make choices in my life that will let me be that way, and because we can't give to someone else what we don't have. That's what a confident goddess is and that's who you have to be.

Why is it so important to love yourself more than anyone else? Because ultimately, we are responsible for our actions and our choices, and the outcome of those actions and choices. So if you go on a date and it doesn't go well and he never texts you again, it doesn't matter because you have confidence in yourself and you love yourself and know what's good about you. You don't need some guy to tell you that. Or if you walk into a new singles event and are out of your comfort zone because you don't know anyone there, it doesn't matter because you know that your best friend is there looking out for you – and that best friend is you.

You know how you treat someone you really care about? The way you love and support that person and treat him or her with kindness and respect? Do that for yourself. And just as you'd challenge a close friend who's making bad decisions about his or her dating life, challenge yourself as well. Just like you would for a good friend, remind yourself over and over again of your immense worth and that you deserve a great man in your life. Challenge yourself to be the best goddess you can be and to meet a great, inspiring man who loves you as much as your best friend does.

When you are your own best friend and are making decisions that are good for you, then you are truly able to go get him. You will do extraordinary things and meet extraordinary men because you will stop looking for validation and for someone to complete you. Now you are in a place where you complete other people.

Support sheet snapshot

Most people have the potential to meet amazing lovers and have great relationships, but potential isn't good enough. Research shows that only 20% of people achieve anything close to their true potential, and this figure is true for dating too. When I work with clients as a coach, we develop a meaningful vision of their dating future and make positive changes in their lives. I help clients to set specific dating goals, then assist them to get over any obstacles in order to develop a focused dating plan of action that gives their dating lives structure and accountability.

The next exercise is an opportunity for you to do the same thing. It's like having your own dating coach or expert by your side. It has been proven that people who visualise themselves attaining their goals and visions have a greater chance of achieving them. By seeing yourself with the man you want and having the relationship you want, you can literally feel your success through your senses, and this increases your power to attract men.

EXERCISE:
SUPPORT SHEET SNAPSHOT

The overall vision I have for my desired dating life:

....

....

....

....

How I most want to feel every day:

....

....

....

....

Things I can do every day to help me stay connected to how I want to feel and to be my goddess self:

....

....

....

....

My greatest dating strengths:

....

....

....

....

....

My biggest dating challenges:

....

....

....

....

My dating mentoring team consists of the following people:

....

....

....

....

....

My short-term dating goals (three months from now):

....

....

....

....

My medium-term dating goals (one year from now):

....

....

....

....

My long-term dating goals (three years from now):

....

....

....

....

❤ ❤ ❤

♥

Getting Fired Up for a First Date

You know what your dating goals are, you've unleashed your inner goddess and you're as fabulous as you can be. Yet there's no getting around the fact that so much depends on those first few minutes when you meet a new person face to face and make your initial impressions. And I'd be lying if I said there wasn't going to be some awkward moments and first date jitters. I did a survey of 100 of my clients a few months ago and nearly a third of the men and women admitted being massively nervous before a first date. Nerves are natural. Rather than delving into the reasons why you're nervous, let's just get straight into sharing a few tricks of the trade with you, which can make all the difference.

First date tips

Steady on

Nerves can actually be healthy! After all, they mean you're excited by the possibilities ahead. They mean you're engaged and interested. They mean you want to make a good impression. These are all terrific things to bring to a first encounter with someone. Oftentimes nerves are nothing more than the usual butterflies. Embrace the butterflies! If your nerves are overwhelming you, you can keep them in check by simply saying to yourself, 'This is not the most useful way for me to feel right now.' Being positive, fun, confident, flirty, open, engaging and a good listener are all useful behaviours on a date. Simply being aware of the fact that you're nervous will allow you to control how you want to come across rather than letting it control you.

Location, location, location

Carefully consider the setting of a first date. Suggest a place or an activity that puts you at ease, not one that makes you feel flustered. Keep it casual and loose instead of elaborate and rigid. Stay away from structured dates or anything too expensive, which puts too much pressure on the date. Don't pick a place where you think all your friends will be hanging out. And don't drink too much. I'm a big fan of going for a casual drink followed by a few light tapas – the conversation starters are in the food. On the first date, it's best to keep it simple and low key.

Shift your perspective

The single best thing you can do to prepare for a first date is to keep a healthy, other-centric perspective. A better, less stressful approach to take is to shift your mental energy and focus on the other person instead of yourself. Try to really listen to every word your date says. Make every effort to really get to know him. Pay attention to all the details – the way he acts, his mannerisms, etc. By shifting the focus onto your date and away from yourself, you'll start to feel more relaxed. Plus you'll also get better insights into whether he has real potential.

Change your tune

Remember the playlist you made on page 186 to get you in the mood for a night out on the town? Turn it on and crank it up when you're getting ready for a first date.

EXERCISE: MAKE THE SPARKS FLY

Try to remember a time when you had loads of chemistry on a date. Imagine you are back on the date. Even if the date wound up being a shambles, it doesn't matter for this exercise – just focus on the chemistry here and try to pinpoint that feeling.

1. How did your body feel?

....

....

2. Where in your body did you feel this?

3. What were you thinking?

4. What did you see?

5. What did you hear?

6. How did you act?

7. Think of a colour to describe the way you were feeling. This will be your chemistry-inducing colour.

Imagine this colour in the body part you listed above in #2. As you take a deep breath, imagine the colour slowly starting to flow throughout your body, flowing down into your legs, touching and tingling your feet, arms, hands and fingertips until you are completely filled with this colour.

Now the next time you go on a date or are flirting with a guy, repeat this exercise, allowing your chemistry colour to slowly build inside of you until it eventually fills you up. How will you act then?

♥ ♥ ♥

First date dos and don'ts

All dating is about finding out whether or not you like a guy. What's wrong with that? When did dating become such a dirty word? When did it become so serious? All the same, there are good ways and bad ways of handling a first date. Coming to town with truckloads of wants is not cool.

Don't talk about marriage or commitment

Don't sit there and talk about how you want to get married and have three kids. Don't even say the words *marriage*, *commitment* or *relationship* at all! Don't think of your date as a potential husband. View him as someone you could go out with again and get to know better.

Don't talk about your need to have kids

The guy will immediately feel like you're just weighing him up as a daddy. He wants to know that you are attracted to him, not just sizing him up as a potential pram pusher. He wants to feel that you're into him for who he is.

Don't talk about money

Keep any worrisome financial situations to yourself. When you tell a guy you're having money trouble, he'll just think that you're looking for someone to bail you out. As for who pays for the date, traditional etiquette still says that the man should pay for the first date. But don't take it for granted that a man is your personal ATM. If he pays for dinner, offer to pay for drinks afterwards.

Don't dump on him

It's not all about you. Don't complain about everything or spend a lot of time making him listen to all your issues and feelings about everything. But if you find yourself chatting away for more than two or three minutes and he hasn't said anything, take his glazed-over expression or his hand reaching for his phone as your cues to close your pucker.

Don't text too much

Keep texting to a minimum. Only use it for arranging meet-ups or sending little flirty messages. Conversations don't flow the same way via text or even email, so it's harder to truly get to know someone and for relationships to blossom. Save your thoughts and feelings for face to face.

Do try to suss him out

Say you went on a job interview and found out that the company was involved in something illegal or was ripping off its customers in some way. Or what if you knew that after you got the job you would have to move to an isolated area for the rest of your life? Or what if you were told that the company had no maternity cover and you could never have kids? How would you feel? Would you just sit there, smile and not say anything? Would you take the job? No, of course not! You would run a mile.

The same goes for dating. On the first date, you are more or less interviewing this man to find out what he wants from life, what he's passionate about and ultimately if you get along well enough to go on a second date.

So try to suss him out. Is he nice to people in general? Does he talk down to the waiter? How he speaks to others is an indication of how he will treat you. Go out with his friends after a few dates and see how he treats them. Do they have fun? Does he try to buy them off? Is he respectful of his friends? Are they laughing and joking with each other? Is he generous and warm with his friends and family?

Do take him at his word

Men are usually pretty direct and will tell you exactly what they're looking for, but many women choose not to listen. For example, if a man tells you that he's just come out of a long-term relationship and isn't looking for anything serious right now, he means it. But a woman hears that and thinks, 'I know he says that he's not looking for anything right now, but I'm going to treat him so good that I'll make him change his mind.' So the next time a man tells you something, listen carefully to what he says. If you want a further explanation, ask him to clarify it or confront him on his bull-shit. This way, you can avoid misunderstandings in the future. No matter how amazing or beautiful or seductive you might be, if a man tells you that he doesn't think he can be in a relationship right now, then you need to respect that. You're not going to change him. Be the flame, give him space and focus on your other dates, and he won't see you as frustrated, upset or delusional. And you never know – you might end up in a relationship with him after all.

Do listen

Sometimes the best thing a woman can do is listen. And when you listen, try to imagine his scenario and focus on his situation, not how his story fits into your own life. So instead of thinking about how a story he tells about work sounds like something that happened at your office, simply try to visualise his story as he tells it. And don't interrupt him with personal-interest triggers like 'That reminds me of the time when', 'That's exactly like when I'. You get the idea. Just let him talk, and remember that listening is critical to love.

Do have fun

At the end of the day, the best advice for a first date is to just have fun. Don't put too much pressure on the situation. Look at the date as an opportunity to have a new experience and meet someone new. You can't control how the other person approaches the date, but you have total control about what you bring to the table.

DateTracker

Set weekly targets and keep yourself on track with the DateTracker. It's not fancy, but I have found that when it comes to dating, the simpler, the better.

As you use your DateTracker, you'll start to see a pattern. It will also identify any areas that could be improved on. How many emails do you need to send to get three dates? How many dates do you need to go on to get one that leads on to a second date? If you find your numbers are low, call your support team. They can review your DateTracker with you and help you figure out which areas you need to improve in. For example, if you're going on loads of first dates but none of them are materialising into a second date, you may need to re-examine how to make a great first impression.

Using your DateTracker is easy – here's how.

- ♥ At the beginning of the week, set targets and write them in the far left column.
- ♥ Track your actions every day. Be honest with yourself.
- ♥ At the end of the week, compare your totals with your targets.
- ♥ Your numbers will tell you a lot about how you're doing.

WEEKLY TARGET	ACTIVITY	MON	TUES
	New prospects from dating networks		
	Emails sent on online dating sites		
	Calls or texts about dating		
	New prospects from friends, family or work		
	New prospects from places I've been		
	Dates I went on		
	Dates moving to date 2		
	Am I living the life of a goddess?		
	How many mentors was I in contact with?		

Getting Fired Up for a First Date

WED	THURS	FRI	SAT	SUN	TOTAL

♥

Keep Your Flame Alive

You've been creating opportunities to meet men and using the *Go Get Him* attitude, and now you've found a guy who you like, gone on over five dates with him and you think there may be a potential relationship there.

So what next? What do you do when you decide to stop dating and start to develop an exclusive relationship with a guy?

Tread carefully and never make it look like you're rushing him down the aisle. But if you're close enough to have sex, you're close enough to ask him what type of relationship you're getting involved in. It seems silly for adults to refer to each other as 'boyfriend' and 'girlfriend', but you need some way to establish what kind of relationship you're in.

Give me a sign

If he hasn't said the words to you just yet and you don't think you have the guts to ask him straight out, there are several ways guys let you know that they want a relationship with you.

1. He consistently prioritises you

Maybe it's planning a weekend away for the two of you, changing his usual Friday night pints with the lads to go to the theatre with you or texting you in the morning to wish you luck in an interview. Whatever it is, it shows he is thinking about you and wants to spend more time with you.

2. He integrates you into his world

Once a guy is ready to be with you, he'll want his friends and family to know about it. Getting you involved with them is his way of saying that you're not just a fling. On the other hand, if he is keen to keep you away at all costs, it might signal that he doesn't want you to get too close so that he can drop you as fast as you came in.

3. He goes out of his way to plan quirky dates

The more effort he puts into planning special dates, the more you know he wants to impress you. If he only plans dates that don't require him to go out of his way – he only asks you to come over to his place or to the pub five minutes down the road – then it's likely this guy only wants you when it's convenient for him.

4. He talks about future plans

If a guy is talking about future events with you in them, then it's a sure sign that he already sees you two together in the future. Be wary, though, if he avoids talking about plans more than a week in advance, if he shifts nervously in his seat when you mention something the two of you might do in the future or if he says things like 'We should have dinner there next time' or 'We'll have more time when work is less busy next month.'

Keep your flame alive

Once the dating dust settles, this is not the time to sit back and let it all hang out. Nor is it the time to rush your man down the aisle just because you're in a relationship. You must remember to continue to be your goddess self, which will help you to keep your flame alive, take care of yourself, avoid destructive patterns and stay simply irresistible to him.

EXERCISE: HAPPILY EVER AFTER

Ask your dating mentors for their best love advice.

1. ....

2. ....

3. ....

4. ....

5. ....

Now come up with one of your own. Write down what you think the secret of love is. Don't be shy! Everyone's definition of love is different. It might well be the secret for your very own happily ever after.

....

....

....

♥ ♥ ♥

Go get him!

Congratulations on getting to the final chapter. What you do now determines any number of possibilities that you can create in your life.

Many people follow the same well-worn path of comfort and repeat the same cycles as dating moths again and again in their lives. But the decision to step outside your front door, to try something new and increase your networks, to use more teasing language to induce chemistry rather than being too nice and to surround yourself with positive influences in your life will all have an effect on where you end up in your life.

Love, opportunities and great men have not left the planet. Your time has come to be the flame and to be your goddess self. Being self-aware, learning and practising the art of creating your own destiny, having the guts to get out of your comfort zone and move away from your destructive dating habits, creating opportunities to meet new people and lovers who will enrich your life, developing and adhering to the principles of a goddess woman and deciding to be the chooser rather than waiting to be chosen will all guarantee that your life is filled with love, fun and adventure. In fact, these choices will improve all areas of your life. Just how far you take these skills is up to you.

If you follow the lessons set out in this book, you'll meet many new and exciting men. But your happiness isn't just about relationships. Regardless of how your own love story plays out, the bottom line is living a dating life that matters to you.

This is your time to go on the adventure of a lifetime: the adventure of the heart. You are an amazing woman with something special that only you are capable of bringing to a man. It's time to become your goddess self. You have the confidence, strength, sexiness and feminine beauty to attract the relationship you deserve. It's time to create your **OTM**s. Make it happen. No more living like a moth. This is your time to shine. You can do it! Applying the lessons in this book will enable you to live a dating life that's so much better than the one you've lived until now. I wish you the very best in your dating journey. Here's to you creating the love you want.

So go on – Go Get Him!

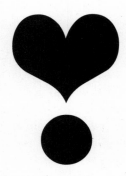